The Simplicity of NATURAL AND HERBAL REMEDIES

A Beginner's Guide to Herbal Medicine

How to Make Teas, Herbal Tinctures, and Salves for Natural Wellness

Joël Beacons

Legal Notice

This book is protected by copyright law and is intended for personal use only. Any unauthorized distribution, modification, reproduction, sale, or use of any part of this book, including quoting or paraphrasing, is strictly prohibited without the prior consent of the author or publisher.

Disclaimer

The information in this book is provided for educational and entertainment purposes only. The author and publisher make no warranties or guarantees of any kind, either expressed or implied, about the accuracy, applicability, or effectiveness of the contents.

The author and ClearPath Publishers LLC expressly disclaim any liability for any damages or losses, whether direct or indirect, that may result from the use or misuse of the information presented herein. Readers are encouraged to consult a licensed medical professional before attempting any techniques outlined in this book. The content is not intended as a substitute for professional advice, and by using this book, readers acknowledge their full responsibility for any decisions regarding their health.

Interior design and print layout by Zakirunissa Karthigeyan.

ISBN: eBook: 978-1-965911-00-6
Paperback: 978-1-965911-01-3
Hardcover: 978-1-965911-02-0

To the remarkable people of Ecuador, whose perseverance through hardship and joyful spirit have taught me the true meaning of patience and the beauty of finding laughter even in challenging times. Your courage and warmth are an endless source of inspiration.

TABLE OF CONTENTS

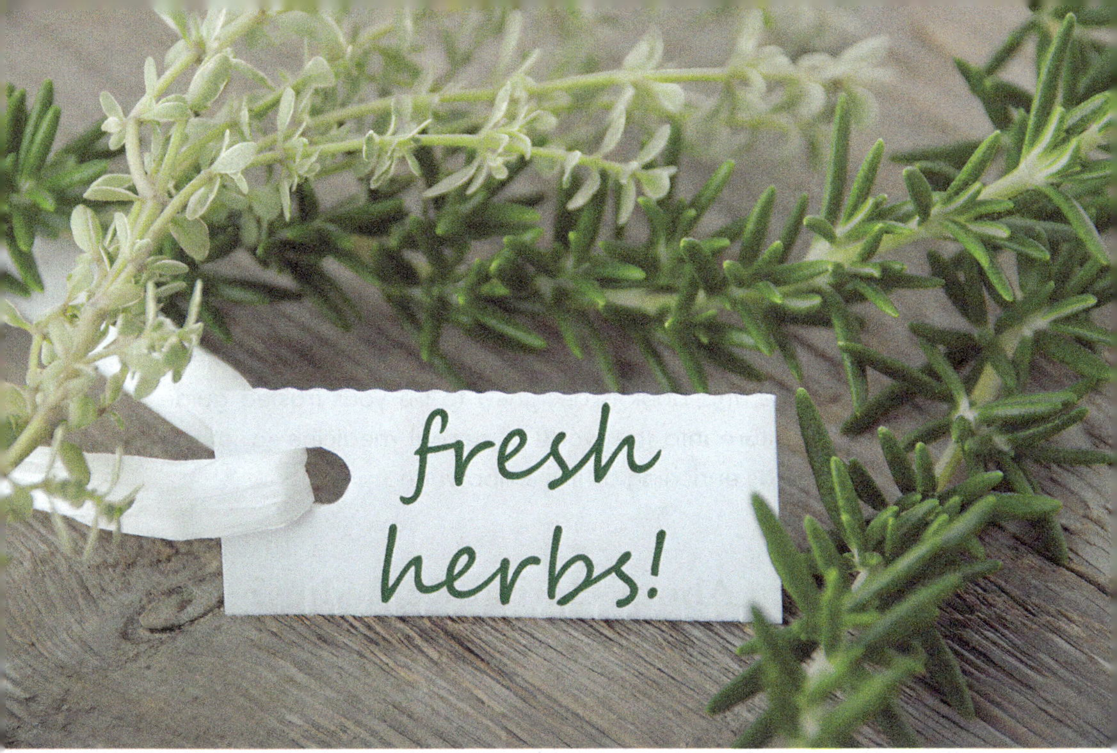

INTRODUCTION

Welcome to a journey that promises to transform your understanding of health, healing, and the power of nature. The purpose of this book is to guide you through the world of herbal remedies in a way that is both thorough and easy to understand. Inside, you'll discover 25 versatile herbs, learn about their use in 10 therapeutic applications, and find 50 practical herbal remedies you can make at home.

In our modern world, where quick fixes and synthetic solutions often dominate healthcare conversations, many of us find ourselves yearning for a more holistic approach to natural wellness. Perhaps you've stood before a pharmacy shelf, overwhelmed by options, wondering if there's a gentler, more sustainable way to support your health. If so, you're not alone.

This book isn't about rejecting modern medicine—far from it. Instead, it's about expanding your herbal medicine toolkit, integrating nature's pharmacy into your wellness routine, and empowering you with knowledge to make informed decisions about your health.

Whether you're looking to address specific health concerns, enhance your overall wellness, or simply connect more deeply with the healing power of nature, this book is designed to be your trusted guide. Let's start this adventure into the world of herbal medicine—a journey that promises to be as enriching as it is empowering.

Why Learn About Herbal Remedies?

There are many reasons why you might have picked up this book; maybe you're

Exploring Complementary Health Approaches: You're interested in exploring natural, holistic ways to support your health and well-being, and you're curious about how herbal remedies can complement your current health practices.

Seeking Reliable, Science-Based Information: You're looking for a trusted resource that provides evidence-based information about herbal remedies, so you can make informed decisions about your health.

Prioritizing Safety and Efficacy: You want to learn how to use herbal remedies safely and effectively, and you're seeking guidance on best practices for selecting, preparing, and using herbs.

Taking an Active Role in Your Health: You're ready to take a proactive, preventative approach to your health, and you're excited to learn how herbal remedies can support your wellness goals.

Embracing Sustainable, Natural Solutions: You're interested in health solutions that are not only good for you but also good for the planet, and you're eager to learn about the sustainability and environmental impact of herbal medicine.

Whatever your reason, it's the perfect time to dive into the world of herbal medicine. The book is designed to assist you in achieving all these goals, equipping you with the necessary knowledge, tools, and inspiration to confidently integrate herbal remedies into your life. As a beginner or experienced herb user, this book will help you achieve natural wellness.

Herbs for Health and Wellness

Typically, we categorize herbs into three main functions or uses. Herbal traditions widely recognize these categories, which guide the use of herbs for health and wellness. The most common categories in traditional herbalism are culinary herbs, aromatic herbs, and medicinal herbs.

Culinary Herbs: These are herbs primarily used in cooking to enhance the flavor of food. However, culinary herbs often have medicinal benefits as well, making them part of both daily meals and healing practices.

- Examples: Rosemary, Garlic, and Turmeric
- Uses: Improve digestion, boost immune function, and add flavor to food

Aromatic Herbs: These herbs are known for their fragrance and often contain volatile oils that are used in herbal medicine, aromatherapy, and personal care products. In addition to their medicinal uses, these herbs' distinctive scent makes them valuable for mood enhancement, stress relief, and emotional wellness.

- Examples: Lavender, Peppermint, Lemon Balm, Chamomile
- Uses: Commonly used in essential oils, inhalations, or as teas to relieve stress, soothe anxiety, or boost the respiratory system

Medicinal Herbs: As the primary focus of this book, these herbs are used primarily for their healing properties. We'll discover that medicinal herbs treat a wide range of health conditions, from acute symptoms like colds or headaches to chronic conditions like arthritis or insomnia.

- Examples: Echinacea, Valerian, St. John's Wort, Elderberry, Astragalus
- Uses: Used in teas, tinctures, salves, and other remedies to support bodily functions and promote healing

What Sets This Book Apart

In a sea of herbal remedy guides, this book stands out for several key reasons:

Curated Selection of Powerhouse Herbs: Instead of overwhelming you with an encyclopedic list, this book focuses on 25 versatile, effective, and accessible herbs. We have carefully selected these herbs based on their therapeutic versatility and ease of use.

Science-Backed Approach: Each herb and remedy is presented with current scientific understanding, helping you grasp not just the "what" but the "why" and "how" of herbal medicine.

Practical, Actionable Advice: This isn't just a book of facts; it's a guide to action. You'll learn how to source, prepare, and use these herbs in your daily life with clear instructions and safety guidelines.

Emphasis on Safety and Integration: This book covers dosage, potential interactions, and precautions. You'll learn how to use herbal remedies safely, including how they can complement conventional treatments.

Sustainability Focus: Explore ethical sourcing and sustainable growing practices, ensuring that your journey into herbal medicine aligns with environmental stewardship.

Personalized Approach: Recognizing that everyone's health journey is unique, this book provides tools to help you tailor herbal remedies to your individual needs and constitution.

Easy-to-Follow Herbal Remedy Recipes: This book is filled with simple, step-by-step instructions for making your own herbal teas, tinctures, and salves, designed to be accessible for beginners.

Gateway to Herbal Medicine: By learning to make your own herbal remedies, you'll gain hands-on experience with the power of plants. This practical experience is often the gateway to a deeper understanding and appreciation of herbal medicine, setting you on the path to becoming a confident and knowledgeable home herbalist.

What's Inside

Here's what to expect as you begin your journey into herbalism:

Foundations of Herbal Medicine: We'll explore the rich history and science behind herbal remedies, giving you a solid understanding of how these natural medicines work in your body.

25 Essential Herbs for 10 Therapeutic Applications: Discover how 25 versatile herbs can support various body systems and address common health concerns. Learn about each herb's properties, uses, and the scientific research supporting their efficacy.

Sourcing and Quality: Learn how to obtain high-quality herbs, whether you're purchasing them or foraging them on your own.

Herb Gardening: Discover how to grow your own medicinal herbs, even in limited spaces, by learning the basics of herb gardening. From choosing the right location to harvesting and storing your homegrown herbs, this section will guide you through the process of cultivating your own herbal medicine supply.

Herbal Preparation Types: Learn the methodology for preparing teas, tinctures, and salves.

50 Herbal Recipes: Explore a range of herbal remedies you can make at home, each designed to support various parts of the body. You'll find clear instructions and dosage guidelines for each recipe.

The Future of Herbalism: We'll look at emerging trends and ongoing research in herbal medicine, keeping you at the forefront of this evolving field.

It's crucial to understand that while herbal remedies can be powerful allies in your health journey, they are not a replacement for professional medical advice, especially for serious conditions. This book emphasizes safe usage, potential interactions with medications, and when it's important to consult with a healthcare provider.

The goal is to empower you with knowledge, enabling you to make informed decisions about integrating herbal remedies into your overall health plan. You'll be provided with the tools to use these natural medicines responsibly and effectively.

The Journey Ahead

As you start this journey, I invite you to approach it with an open mind and a critical eye. Question, explore, and most importantly, listen to your body. Preparing herbal remedies is as much an art as it is a science, and your own experiences will be an important part of your learning process.

CHAPTER 1:
FOUNDATIONS OF HERBAL MEDICINE

The world of herbal medicine is a fascinating blend of ancient wisdom and modern science. This chapter will take you on a journey through time, exploring the rich history of herbal remedies and their evolution into contemporary practice. We'll delve into the core principles of herbalism, uncover how these natural medicines work in your body, and lay the groundwork for safe, effective use of herbal remedies.

Ancient Remedies and Rich Traditions

Herbal medicine has been an integral part of human health practices for millennia. Its roots stretch back to the very dawn of human civilization, with evidence of herbal use dating back over 60,000 years. This long history is not just a testament to tradition, but to the enduring efficacy of plant-based remedies.

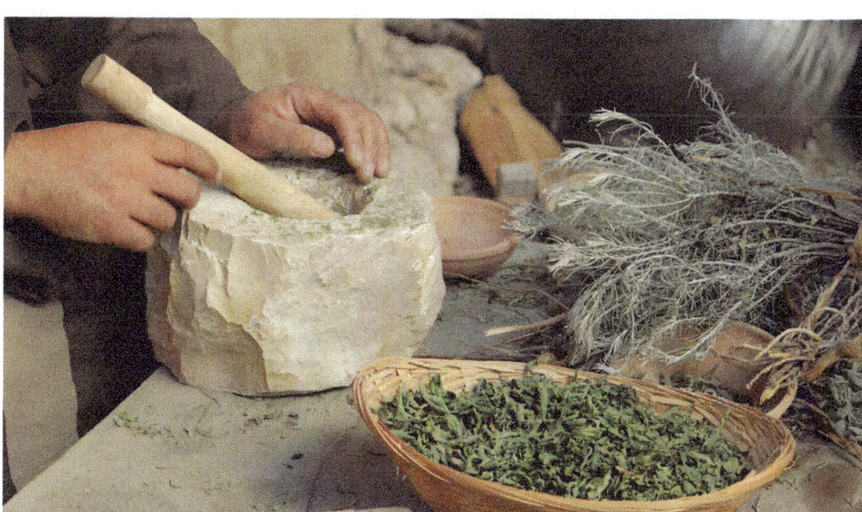

Ancient Egypt

In ancient Egypt, around 1500 B.C.E., the Ebers Papyrus documented over 850 herbal medicines (Metwaly et al., 2021). This comprehensive medical text demonstrates the sophisticated understanding of herbal remedies in one of the world's earliest civilizations. Modern scientific research validates the continued use of many ancient Egyptian remedies, such as Garlic for heart health and Aloe Vera for skin conditions, today. Researchers have extensively researched the cardiovascular and immune-supporting benefits of Garlic, which ancient Egyptians and many other cultures used medicinally.

Traditional Chinese Medicine

Across the globe, in ancient China, the development of Traditional Chinese Medicine (TCM) was underway. The "Shennong Ben Cao Jing," or "The Divine Farmer's Materia Medica," compiled around the year 200 BC, detailed 365 medicines derived from minerals, plants, and animals (Wilms, 2017). TCM's holistic approach to health, emphasizing balance and prevention, continues to influence modern integrative medicine practices.

Ayurvedic Tradition

In India, the Ayurvedic tradition, dating back to around the year 400, developed a complex system of diagnosis and herbal treatment (Pandey et al., 2013). Ayurveda's emphasis on individualized treatment plans based on a person's unique constitution aligns remarkably well with modern personalized medicine approaches. Studies have demonstrated the powerful anti-inflammatory and antioxidant properties of Turmeric, a staple in Ayurvedic medicine.

Native American Herbal Traditions

Native American tribes across North and South America developed their own rich traditions of herbal medicine, often intertwining physical healing with spiritual practices. Many of these traditions emphasize the interconnectedness of human health with the natural world, a perspective increasingly validated by modern ecological and medical research. Native American tribes use Echinacea for various ailments, and researchers have studied its potential to support immune function (Borchers et al., 2000).

European Herbal Traditions

European herbal traditions, influenced by Greek and Roman medical knowledge, evolved through the Middle Ages and Renaissance. The work of herbalists like Nicholas Culpeper in the 17th century laid the groundwork for modern Western herbal medicine. Chamomile, utilized for centuries in European and Middle Eastern traditional medicine, has been the subject of multiple studies examining its calming and digestive health properties (Dai et al., 2022).

This rich global history of herbal medicine is not merely of academic interest. Many of these ancient remedies have stood the test of time and scientific scrutiny. Understanding this historical context provides valuable insights into the potential of herbal remedies and the importance of the holistic, preventative approach often emphasized in traditional herbal practices.

Herbalism as Integrative Medicine

While the roots of herbal healing stretch deep into our past, its branches extend firmly into our present and future. The last few decades have seen a remarkable shift in how the scientific and medical communities view herbalism.

No longer dismissed as mere folklore, many herbal remedies are now the subject of rigorous scientific study. Advanced analytical techniques allow us to identify and study the active compounds in medicinal plants, while controlled clinical trials help us understand their effects on human health. This scientific approach has led to some remarkable discoveries and validations:

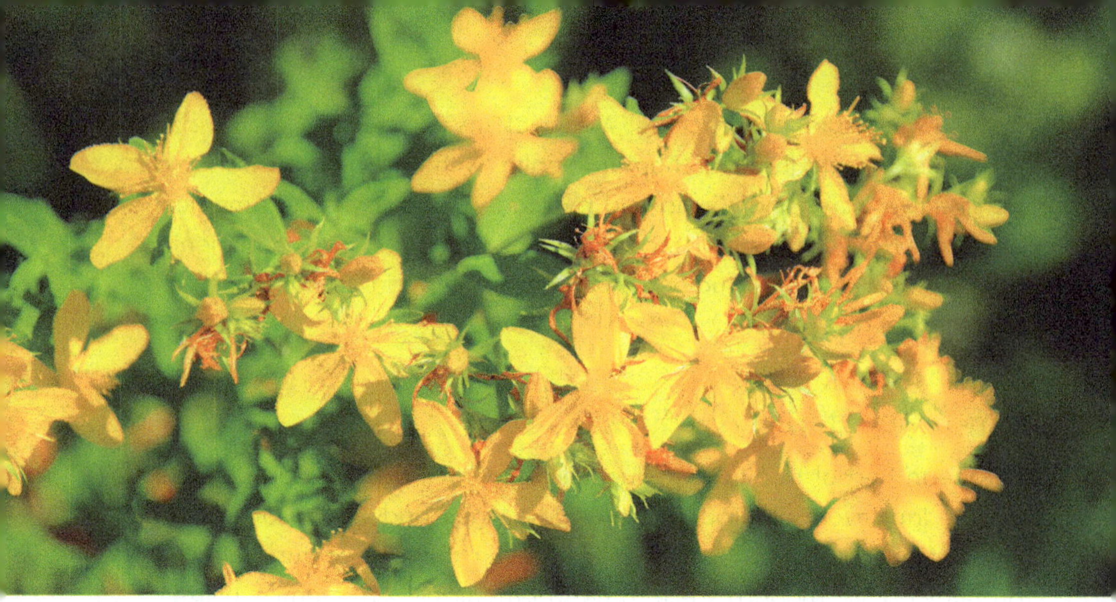

St. John's Wort (*Hypericum perforatum*), traditionally used for mood disorders, has been shown in multiple clinical trials to be effective for mild to moderate depression. A Cochrane review found it to be as effective as standard antidepressants for major depression, with fewer side effects (Linde et al., 2008).

Ginger (*Zingiber officinale*), long used for digestive issues, has been validated through clinical research for its antiemetic properties. It's now recommended by some oncology departments for chemotherapy-induced nausea (Ryan et al., 2011).

Advancements in pharmacognosy (the study of medicines derived from natural sources) are helping us understand the complex ways in which herbal remedies interact with our bodies (Pan et al., 2014). We're discovering that many herbs contain multiple active compounds that work synergistically, often providing benefits that isolated compounds cannot match (Williamson, 2001).

This blend of traditional knowledge and scientific inquiry is fostering a more integrative approach to healthcare. Many medical institutions now offer integrative medicine programs that combine conventional treatments with evidence-based complementary therapies, including herbal medicine (Coulter et al., 2013).

The modern perspective on herbal medicine also emphasizes safety and quality control. Ekor (2013) emphasizes the need for standardization of herbal products, rigorous testing for contaminants, and research into herb-drug interactions to ensure the safe and effective use of herbal medicines alongside conventional treatments.

As we face global health challenges and a growing need for sustainable healthcare practices, herbal medicine, with its emphasis on plant-based remedies and traditional ecological knowledge, is well-positioned to contribute to more sustainable, accessible health solutions.

Terminology

Before diving into the principles and practices of herbal medicine, it's essential to understand some basic terminology. These terms form the foundation of how herbalists describe the properties and effects of different herbs, and understanding them will help you better grasp the therapeutic uses and potential benefits of various plants:

Actions: In herbal medicine, "actions" refer to the specific physiological effects that an herb has on the body. These actions describe how the herb interacts with different systems or processes in the body, such as digestion, circulation, or the immune system. Understanding an herb's actions can help you choose the most appropriate plants for specific health concerns and create targeted herbal formulas. Some common herbal actions include:

- Anti-inflammatory: Reduces inflammation in the body
- Diuretic: Increases urine production and helps eliminate excess fluid
- Expectorant: Helps expel mucus from the lungs and airways
- Carminative: Relieves gas and bloating in the digestive system

- Adaptogen: Helps the body adapt to stress and promotes overall balance

Energetics: Energetics is a traditional way of describing the properties of herbs based on their effects on the body's temperature, moisture, and overall balance. This system originated in ancient healing traditions, such as Ayurveda and TCM, but has been adapted by Western herbalists as well (Niemeyer et al., 2013). By understanding an herb's energetics, herbalists can select plants that help restore balance in the body and address the root cause of health issues rather than just treating symptoms. The main energetic qualities include:

- Temperature: Herbs can be described as warming (stimulating and increasing circulation) or cooling (calming and reducing inflammation).
- Moisture: Herbs can be either moistening (adding moisture to the body) or drying (helping to eliminate excess moisture).
- Tone: Some herbs are considered relaxing (promoting relaxation and reducing tension), while others are stimulating (increasing energy and promoting circulation).

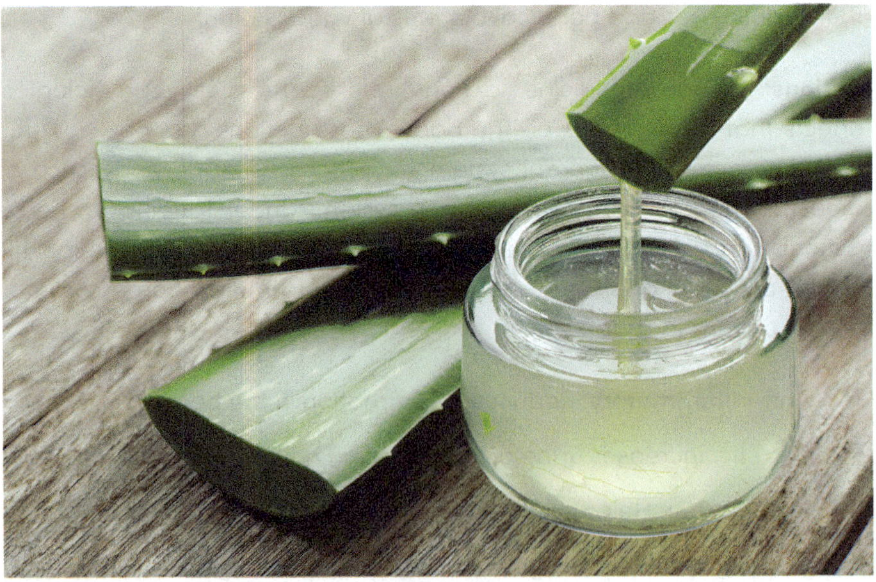

Adaptogen: Adaptogens are a unique class of herbs that help the body adapt to stress and promote overall balance. These herbs work by regulating the body's stress response, supporting the adrenal glands, and promoting homeostasis (a state of internal stability and balance). Adaptogens are commonly used to help manage stress, improve resilience, and support overall well-being. They are generally safe for long-term use and can be incorporated into daily wellness routines (Panossian & Wikman, 2010). Some well-known adaptogens include:

- Ashwagandha (*Withania somnifera*)
- Rhodiola (*Rhodiola rosea*)
- Holy Basil (*Ocimum sanctum*)
- Ginseng (*Panax ginseng*)

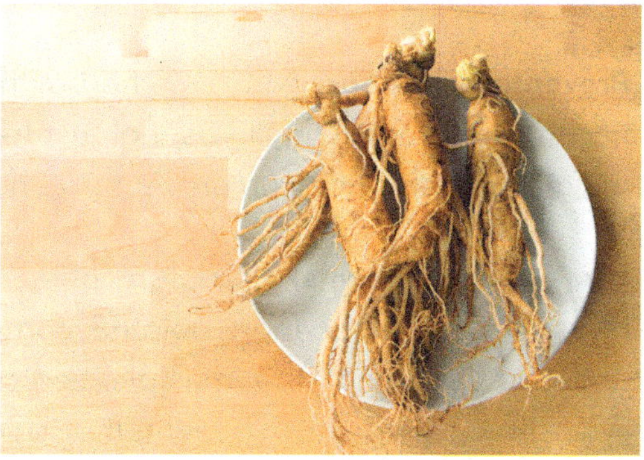

By familiarizing yourself with these key terms, you'll be better equipped to understand the properties and potential benefits of different herbs, and how they can be used to support health and well-being. As you continue to learn about herbal medicine, you'll encounter many more specific terms related to plant chemistry, herbal preparation methods, and therapeutic applications. However, understanding actions, energetics, and adaptogens provides a solid foundation for your herbal studies.

Herbalism: A Holistic Approach to Health

Herbalism is more than just the use of plants for medicinal purposes. It's a comprehensive approach to health and wellness that considers the whole person—body, mind, and spirit—in the context of their environment.

At its core, herbalism is about supporting the body's innate ability to heal and maintain balance. Rather than simply treating symptoms, herbalism seeks to address the root causes of health issues and support overall wellness (Bone & Mills, 2013).

Key aspects of herbalism include (*Sustainable Herbs Initiative*, n.d.):

Holistic Perspective: Herbalism views health issues not as isolated problems, but as indications of imbalance in the whole system. A headache, for instance, might be seen not just as pain in the head, but potentially as a sign of stress, hormonal imbalance, or digestive issues.

Individuality: Herbal approaches are tailored to the individual. What works for one person with similar symptoms may not work for another. This personalized approach aligns with the growing trend towards precision medicine in conventional healthcare.

Preventative Focus: Much of herbal medicine is about maintaining health and preventing illness, not just treating disease. This aligns with the growing emphasis on preventative health in modern medicine.

Use of Whole Plants: Herbalism often favors the use of whole plant preparations rather than isolated compounds. This is based on the understanding that the multiple compounds in a plant often work synergistically, providing benefits that isolated compounds cannot match.

Sustainability: Many herbalists emphasize the importance of sustainable harvesting and cultivation practices, recognizing the interconnectedness of human and environmental health. Sustainable herbalism seeks to protect medicinal plants and their ecosystems by promoting ethical wildcrafting, organic cultivation, and conservation efforts to ensure that future generations can benefit from these valuable natural resources.

Herbalism isn't about rejecting modern medicine. Instead, it offers complementary approaches that can work alongside conventional treatments. Many herbalists collaborate with conventional healthcare providers to create integrative treatment plans that leverage the strengths of both approaches.

Herbal Misconceptions

There are several common misconceptions about herbal medicine that need to be addressed:

1. **"Natural" means "safe:"** While herbs are natural substances, they can still have potent effects on the body. Some herbs can cause side effects, interact with medications, or be unsafe for certain individuals. It's important to respect the power of herbs and to use them responsibly.

2. **Herbs are not as effective as conventional drugs:** Many people believe that because herbs are natural, they must be less potent than pharmaceutical drugs. However, plant compounds are the source of many of our modern medicines. Scientific research has validated the effectiveness of herbs when used appropriately

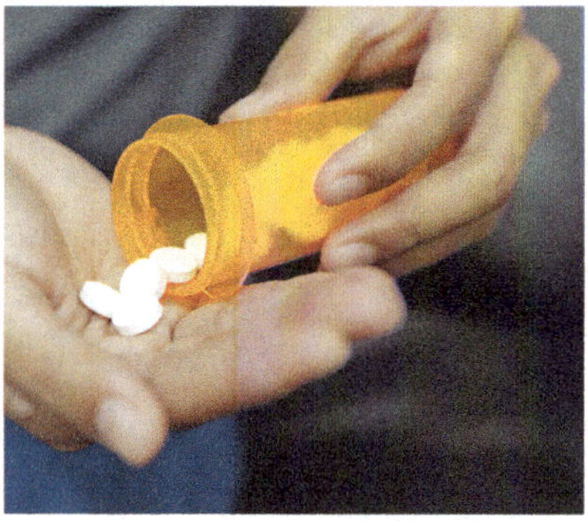

3. **Herbs can replace conventional treatment:** While herbs can be powerful allies in health, they should not be seen as a substitute for necessary medical care. Herbs can complement conventional treatment, but it's important to work with healthcare professionals, especially for serious health conditions.

By understanding and addressing these misconceptions, we can promote a more accurate and responsible understanding of herbal medicine.

How Herbal Remedies Work

Understanding how herbal remedies work involves delving into the complex world of plant biochemistry and human physiology. Herbs contain a vast array of bioactive compounds that can interact with our bodies in myriad ways (Efferth & Koch, 2011).

Let's explore the key concepts:

1. **Phytochemicals—The Power of Plant Compounds:** Phytochemicals are biologically active compounds produced by plants (Wang et al., 2014).
2. **Synergy—The Whole is Greater Than the Sum of Its Parts:** Herbal medicines often work through synergistic effects, where multiple phytochemicals in a plant work together to produce an effect greater than any single phytochemical alone. This synergy can enhance the potency of active phytochemicals, reduce side effects, and provide multiple therapeutic actions simultaneously (Williamson, 2001).
3. **Bioavailability and Absorption:** The effectiveness of herbal remedies depends not just on their active phytochemicals but also on how well these phytochemicals are absorbed and utilized by the body. Factors affecting this include the form of the herb (e.g., tea, tincture, capsule), the presence of other substances that enhance absorption, and individual variations in metabolism and gut health (Zhou et al., 2004).
4. **Interaction With Body Systems:** Herbal remedies can interact with various body systems, including the nervous, immune, endocrine, digestive, and many others. Each herb has specific actions on different systems, which can be harnessed to support overall health and address-specific concerns (Bone & Mills, 2013).
5. **Adaptogenic Effects:** Adaptogens help the body resist stressors of all kinds, whether physical, chemical, or biological (Panossian & Wikman, 2010).
6. **Cumulative and Tonic Effects:** Many herbs work best when taken consistently over time, gradually nudging the body towards balance. This is in contrast to the often immediate but short-lived effects of many pharmaceutical drugs (Bone & Mills, 2013).

By targeting specific body systems with appropriate herbal remedies, herbalists aim to restore balance and support the body's natural healing processes. However, it's crucial to remember that herbs can have complex and wide-ranging effects, often influencing multiple systems simultaneously. This is why a holistic approach, considering the entire person and their unique constitution, is essential in herbal medicine (Foster & Johnson, 2006).

Understanding these mechanisms helps us appreciate the complexity and potential of herbal medicines. It also underscores the importance of using herbs knowledgeably and respecting their power as medicinal agents.

Dosage, Side Effects, and Professional Guidance

While herbal remedies can be powerful in maintaining and restoring health, it's crucial to approach their use with knowledge and caution. Safety is paramount in herbal medicine, just as it is in conventional medicine. Below are essential safety considerations to keep in mind when working with herbal remedies:

1. **The Herbal Safety Continuum Scale:** Herbs can be classified on a safety scale, ranging from safe for general use to toxic. The Herbal Academy has shared the Herbal Safety Continuum Scale, which categorizes herbs into six safety classes based on their potential risks and benefits. For more information on this scale and how to use it, refer to the Herbal Academy's blog post: *www.theherbalacademy.com/blog/the-herb-safety-continuum-scale/*

2. **Potential Side Effects:** Like any active substance, herbs can have side effects. These are often mild but can be serious in some cases (Bent & Ko, 2004).

   - Allergic Reactions: Certain herbs may trigger allergic reactions in some individuals.

   - Herb-Drug Interactions: Some herbs can interact with pharmaceutical drugs, either enhancing or diminishing their effects.

- Quality and Contamination: Ensuring the quality and purity of herbal products is crucial.

3. **Dosage:** The principle of "more is better" does not apply to herbal medicine (Bone & Mills, 2013). Appropriate dosage depends on various factors:
   - The specific herb and its potency
   - The individual's age, weight, and overall health
   - The condition being addressed
   - The form of the herb (e.g., tea, tincture, capsule)
4. **Integration With Conventional Medicine:** Herbal medicine can often complement conventional treatments, but this integration must be managed carefully (Ekor, 2013).
   - Always let healthcare providers know if you're using any herbs or supplements.
   - Be aware of potential interactions between herbs and prescribed medications.
   - Certain medical conditions or treatments may contraindicate the use of herbs in certain cases.

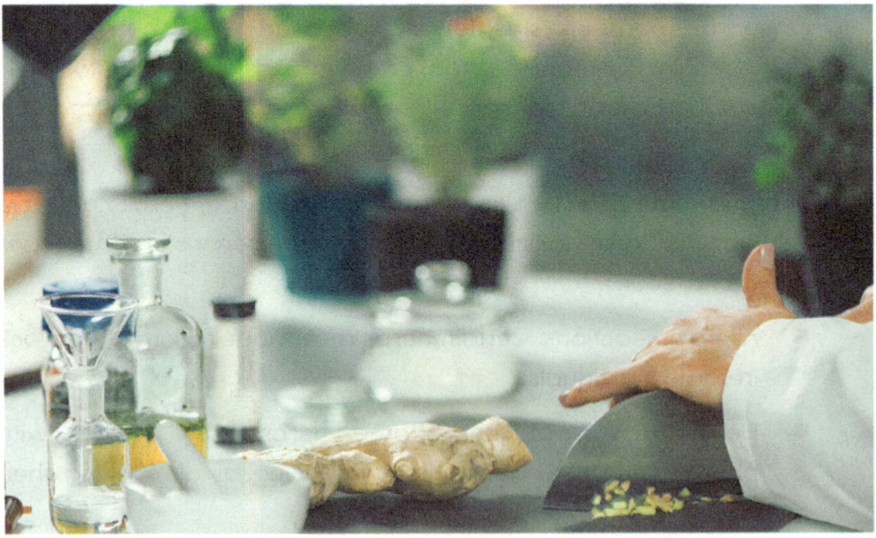

The Importance of Professional Guidance: While many herbs can be safely used for self-care, working with a qualified herbalist or integrative healthcare provider is advisable, especially for complex health issues or when using potent herbs.

By understanding these aspects of herbal medicine, we can harness the power of plants for healing while ensuring safety and efficacy.

Embracing a Holistic Approach to Health

As we conclude this exploration of the foundations of herbal medicine, it's clear that herbalism offers a rich, nuanced approach to health and healing by blending ancient remedies with modern scientific understanding. The journey into herbal medicine is one of continuous learning, self-discovery, and taking an active role in our own well-being. As you continue through this book, you'll gain practical knowledge about specific herbs and their applications, always grounded in the principles of supporting long-term health and balance through a deeper connection to the healing power of nature.

CHAPTER 2:

ESSENTIAL HEALING HERBS

In the world of medicinal plants, choosing which herbs to focus on can be overwhelming. This chapter introduces you to 25 practical medicinal herbs that form the core of this book. We have carefully selected these plants based on specific criteria to ensure their versatility, accessibility, and safety for home use. The herbs featured in this book were chosen based on the following criteria:

Therapeutic Versatility: Each herb offers multiple health benefits and can be used to address various conditions. For example, Ashwagandha is known for its adaptogenic properties, helping the body cope with stress, but it also has anti-inflammatory, sleep-promoting, and immune-boosting effects.

Safety Profile: These herbs have a history of safe use and are generally well-tolerated when used appropriately. However, it's important to note that even safe herbs can have potential side effects or interactions, which is why we emphasize the importance of proper dosage and consultation with healthcare professionals.

Accessibility: All of these herbs are widely available, either through cultivation, ethical wildcrafting, or purchase from reputable suppliers (see the **Resources** section at the end of the book). Many of these herbs, such as Dandelion and Peppermint, can be easily grown in home gardens or found in the wild.

Ease of Use: These herbs can be prepared and used at home without specialized equipment or extensive training. Most of the preparations in this book, such as teas, tinctures, and salves, can be made with simple kitchen tools and basic techniques.

Scientific Backing: While respecting traditional knowledge, we've prioritized herbs with a growing body of scientific research supporting their efficacy. For instance, numerous studies have investigated the anti-inflammatory and pain-relieving properties of Turmeric.

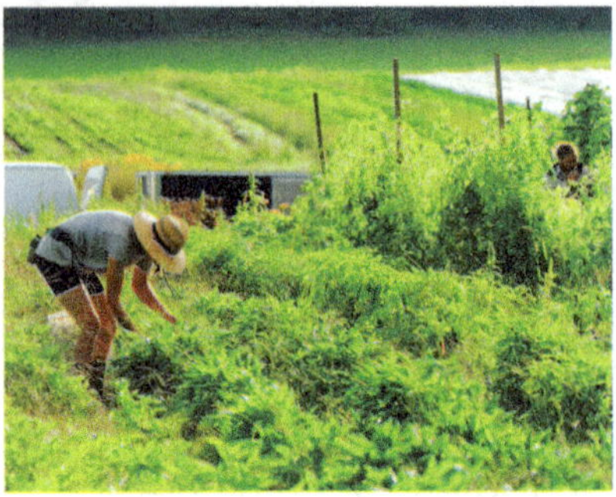

Sustainability: We've considered the environmental impact of not just wildcrafting and growing your own herbs, but the entire supply chain as well. We've included **resources** at the end of this book to learn more about sustainable herbs and recommended suppliers. Sustainable practices aim to ensure that medicinal plants are harvested in ways that do not harm the ecosystems from which they come, while also supporting the communities that depend on them for livelihoods. Ethical wildcrafting, habitat conservation, and organic farming methods are emphasized to protect biodiversity and maintain the long-term health of the environment (*Sustainable Herbs Initiative*, n.d.).

Cultural Significance: Many of these herbs have rich histories in various healing traditions, offering a connection to ancestral wisdom. Herbs like Holy Basil in Ayurvedic medicine and Ginger in TCM have been revered for their medicinal properties for centuries.

By focusing on herbs that meet these criteria, we ensure that you're working with plants that are not only potent and effective but also practical for home use.

Practical Medicinal Herbs

These versatile, easily accessible herbs can be transformed into powerful herbal remedies that can be customized to meet an individual's unique needs. More detailed information on each of these herbs such as botanical information, plant parts used for herbal remedies, dosage guidelines, and contraindications, among other things, can be found in Appendix I: Plant Monographs.

The Herbs Addressed Here Include:

1. **Aloe Vera** (*Aloe barbadensis miller*): immune system support, digestive system support, skin, hair, and beauty, pain management and inflammation.
2. **Ashwagandha** (*Withania somnifera*): stress and anxiety reduction, sleep support and relaxation, cognitive function and memory support, pain management and inflammation, immune system support, women's health.
3. **Astragalus** (*Astragalus membranaceus*): immune system support, energy and vitality enhancement, detoxification, cleanse, and urinary tract support, stress and anxiety reduction.
4. **Burdock** (*Arctium lappa*): skin, hair, and beauty, detoxification, cleanse, and urinary tract support, digestive system support.
5. **Calendula** (*Calendula officinalis*): skin, hair, and beauty, women's health, pain management and inflammation, detoxification, cleanse, and urinary tract support.
6. **Chamomile** (*Matricaria chamomilla*): pain management and inflammation, digestive system support, skin, hair, and beauty, stress and anxiety reduction, sleep support and relaxation, women's health.
7. **Dandelion** (*Taraxacum officinale*): digestive system support, detoxification, cleanse, and urinary tract support.
8. **Echinacea** (*Echinacea purpurea*): immune system support, pain management and inflammation.
9. **Elderberry** (*Sambucus nigra*): immune system support.
10. **Fennel** (*Foeniculum vulgare*): digestive system support, women's health.
11. **Ginger** (*Zingiber officinale*): immune system support, digestive system support, detoxification, cleanse, and urinary tract support, pain management and inflammation.

12. **Goldenseal** (*Hydrastis canadensis*): digestive system support, immune system support, detoxification, cleanse, and urinary tract support.
13. **Holy Basil** (*Ocimum sanctum*): digestive system support, stress and anxiety reduction, immune system support, cognitive function and memory support, pain management and inflammation.
14. **Hops** (*Humulus lupulus*): pain management and inflammation, stress and anxiety reduction, sleep support and relaxation, women's health.
15. **Lavender** (*Lavandula angustifolia*): stress and anxiety reduction, sleep support and relaxation, immune system support, digestive system support.
16. **Lemon Balm** (*Melissa officinalis*): digestive system support, stress and anxiety reduction, sleep support and relaxation, cognitive function and memory support, immune system support.
17. **Licorice** (*Glycyrrhiza glabra*): pain management and inflammation, digestive system support, energy and vitality enhancement, immune system support.
18. **Nettle** (*Urtica dioica*): detoxification, cleanse, and urinary tract support, immune system support, pain management and inflammation, skin, hair, and beauty, women's health.
19. **Passionflower** (*Passiflora incarnata*): sleep support and relaxation, stress and anxiety reduction, cognitive function and memory support.
20. **Peppermint** (*Mentha × piperita*): digestive system support, immune system support, cognitive function and memory support, pain management and inflammation, skin, hair, and beauty.
21. **Rhodiola** (*Rhodiola rosea*): stress and anxiety reduction, energy and vitality enhancement, cognitive function and memory support, immune system support.

22. **Rosemary** (*Rosmarinus officinalis*): digestive system support, pain management and inflammation, detoxification, cleanse, and urinary tract support, cognitive function and memory support, skin, hair, and beauty.
23. **St. John's Wort** (*Hypericum perforatum*): pain management and inflammation, immune system support, digestive system support, women's health, skin, hair, and beauty, stress and anxiety reduction, cognitive function and memory support.
24. **Turmeric** (*Curcuma longa*): pain management and inflammation, cognitive function and memory support, digestive system support, immune system support, detoxification, cleanse, and urinary tract support.
25. **Valerian** (*Valeriana officinalis*): sleep support and relaxation, stress and anxiety reduction.

Each of these herbs has a unique profile of benefits, applications, and preparation methods. In the following chapters, we'll explore how to source, prepare, and use these herbs effectively and safely.

Therapeutic Applications

The 25 herbs indicated above have been selected to support a wide range of body parts and systems. Here's a closer look at each application:

1. **Immune System Support:** Herbs like Echinacea, Elderberry, and Astragalus increase the activity of immune cells, such as natural killer cells and macrophages, and enhance the production of immune-regulating compounds, such as interferon.
2. **Cognitive Function and Memory Support:** Herbs like Rosemary, Holy Basil, and Lemon Balm enhance mental clarity, improve memory, and support overall brain function.
3. **Detoxification, Cleanse, and Urinary Tract Support:** Herbs like Burdock, Dandelion, and Nettle support liver function, stimulate bile production, and enhance the body's natural detoxification processes.

4. **Digestive System Support:** Herbs like Peppermint, Fennel, and Ginger relax digestive muscles, stimulate digestive secretions, and reduce inflammation in the digestive tract.

5. **Energy and Vitality Enhancement:** Herbs like Ashwagandha, Rhodiola, and Holy Basil support energy production, reduce fatigue, and enhance physical and mental endurance.

6. **Pain Management and Inflammation:** Herbs like Turmeric, Ginger, and Nettle reduce inflammation, provide pain relief, and support the body's natural healing processes.

7. **Skin, Hair, and Beauty:** Herbs like Calendula, Aloe Vera, and Lavender support skin healing, promote hair growth, and provide nutrients for skin and hair health.

8. **Sleep Support and Relaxation:** Herbs like Valerian, Passionflower, and Hops increase calming neurotransmitters, promote relaxation, and support healthy sleep patterns.

9. **Stress and Anxiety Reduction:** Herbs like Ashwagandha, Holy Basil, and Lemon Balm regulate stress responses, support adrenal function, and promote mental calmness.

10. **Women's Health:** Herbs like Fennel, Licorice, and St. John's Wort support hormonal balance, ease menstrual discomfort, and help manage menopausal symptoms.

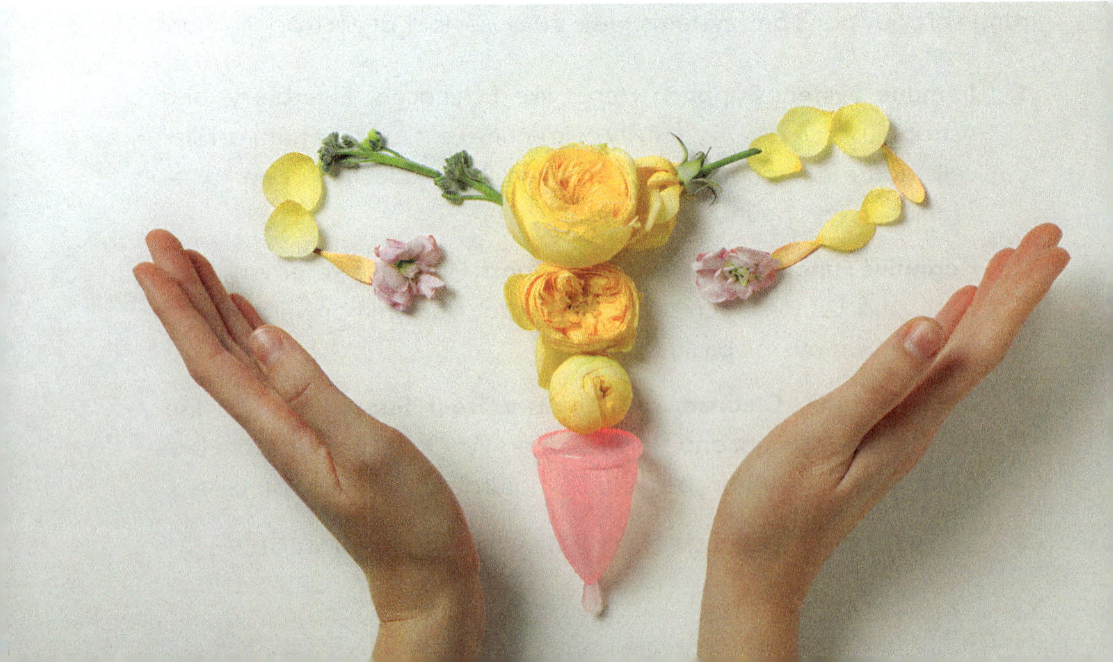

The Power of Plant Allies

These carefully selected herbs offer a remarkably wide range of therapeutic applications. By focusing on a limited number of herbs, you'll have the opportunity to learn the basics of making herbal remedies, practice your skills, and develop a deep, personal relationship with each plant.

As you progress through this book, you'll learn not just about each herb individually, but also how they can work synergistically. You'll discover how to combine these herbs to create personalized, effective herbal remedies tailored to your specific holistic health goals.

Remember, the journey into herbal medicine is one of continuous learning and discovery. These essential herbs are your starting point, your foundation. As you develop a deeper relationship with these plants, you may find yourself naturally expanding your herbal repertoire. But for now, let's begin by getting to know these powerful plant allies.

CHAPTER 3: SOURCING HIGH-QUALITY HERBS

In the realm of herbal medicine, the journey from plant to remedy is as crucial as the remedy itself. This chapter will guide you through the critical process of sourcing high-quality herbs, a skill that forms the foundation of effective and safe herbal practice. Whether you are herb gardening, purchasing from suppliers, or venturing into ethical wildcrafting, the knowledge you gain here will empower you to make informed decisions about the herbs you use.

The Importance of Quality in Herbal Medicine

The efficacy of herbal remedies hinges on the quality of the plants used. Unlike standardized pharmaceutical drugs, herbs are complex natural products whose therapeutic properties can vary widely based on numerous factors. Understanding these factors is crucial for anyone serious about harnessing the full potential of herbal medicine.

Before we jump into the specifics of sourcing, let's explore the key elements that influence herb quality. Each of these factors plays a vital role in determining the potency, safety, and overall effectiveness of your herbal preparations.

1. **Growing Conditions:** Soil quality, climate, and farming practices all influence the plant's chemical composition.
2. **Harvesting Methods:** The time of harvest and the parts of the plant collected can significantly impact potency.
3. **Processing and Storage:** Improper drying, processing, or storage can degrade the active compounds in herbs.

4. **Contamination:** If not grown and handled properly, pesticides, heavy metals, or microorganisms can contaminate herbs.
5. **Adulteration:** Unfortunately, some suppliers may adulterate herbs with cheaper materials to cut costs.

By considering these factors in your sourcing decisions, you lay the groundwork for creating potent and safe herbal remedies. Recall that the quality of your herbs serves as the cornerstone for all your herbal preparations. In the following sections, we'll explore practical strategies for ensuring you obtain the highest quality herbs possible, whether through careful purchasing or ethical wildcrafting.

Accurate Plant Identification

In the world of herbs, a case of mistaken identity can be more than just a simple error—it can be dangerous. Proper identification is not just about finding the right herb; it's about ensuring safety, efficacy, and environmental stewardship. This section will equip you with the knowledge and strategies to confidently identify the herbs you seek to use. For those looking to deepen their identification skills further, be sure to consult the **Resources** section at the end of this book, which lists additional websites and mobile apps dedicated to plant identification. These tools can be invaluable companions in your journey to become proficient in herb identification.

The Risks of Misidentification

Before we dive into identification techniques, it's crucial to understand what's at stake. Misidentification can lead to a range of problems, from ineffective treatments to serious health risks. Here are the key risks to keep in mind:

- **Ineffective Treatment:** Using the wrong herb means you won't get the intended therapeutic effect.

- **Toxicity:** Some plants are toxic and can cause serious harm if ingested or used topically.
- **Endangered Species:** Mistakenly harvesting endangered plants can result in further decline of the population.
- **Legal Issues:** Laws protect some plants and harvesting them may result in legal penalties.

These risks underscore the importance of developing strong identification skills. Whether you're wildcrafting or verifying purchased herbs, accurate identification is your first line of defense against potential dangers and disappointments in your herbal practice.

Plant Identification Strategies

Now that we understand the importance of proper identification, let's explore a comprehensive set of strategies to help you confidently identify herbs. These techniques, when used in combination, will significantly increase your accuracy.

- **Consult Multiple Sources:** Use at least two reliable field guides specific to your region.
- **Learn Botanical Terms:** Understanding basic botanical terminology will help you make sense of plant descriptions in field guides.
- **Use All Your Senses:** Look at the plant's overall form, leaf shape, flower structure, and bark texture.
- **Observe the Plant in Different Seasons:** Many plants look different throughout their growth cycle.
- **Take Clear Photos:** Photograph the whole plant, as well as close-ups of leaves, flowers, and any distinctive features.
- **Seek Expert Guidance:** Consider taking classes or going on plant walks led by experienced herbalists or botanists.

- **Use Technology Wisely:** While plant identification apps can be helpful tools, they should never be your sole method of identification.

By incorporating these strategies into your practice, you'll develop a well-rounded approach to plant identification. Remember, becoming proficient in identification is a journey, not a destination. Each time you practice these techniques, you're building a valuable skill that will serve you throughout your herbal career.

What to Look for When Purchasing Herbs

While growing or foraging your own herbs can be rewarding, purchasing herbs from reputable suppliers is often the most accessible and practical way to source high-quality plant materials. However, not all suppliers are equal, and understanding what to look for can significantly impact the quality of your herbs. In this section, we'll explore the key factors to consider when purchasing herbs, empowering you to make informed decisions and ensuring you're getting the best possible materials for your herbal practice.

Before we dive into the specific criteria, it's important to understand that purchasing herbs is not just a transaction—it's an opportunity to build relationships with suppliers, support sustainable practices, and contribute to the overall quality of the herbal industry. By being a discerning consumer, you not only ensure the efficacy of your own remedies but also encourage higher standards across the board.

Here are the essential factors to consider when purchasing herbs:

- **Organic Certification:** Opt for certified organic herbs whenever possible. Organic certification ensures that the herbs are grown without synthetic pesticides or fertilizers, reducing the risk of harmful residues. While certified organic herbs are ideal, some small-scale growers may follow organic practices without official certification due to the costs involved. In such cases, don't hesitate to ask about their growing methods. Building a relationship with your suppliers can provide valuable insights into their practices and the quality of their products.

- **Proper Storage and Packaging:** High-quality dried herbs should be stored in airtight containers away from light, heat, and moisture. Look for suppliers who use opaque or dark glass containers for light-sensitive herbs.
- **Whole vs. Powdered Herbs:** When possible, choose whole herbs over pre-powdered ones. Whole herbs retain their volatile oils and active compounds longer than powdered herbs.
- **Appearance, Smell, and Taste:** Quality herbs should have a vibrant color close to that of the fresh plant. They should have a strong, characteristic aroma and taste.
- **Correct Plant Parts:** Ensure you're getting the correct part of the plant for your intended use. Different parts of a plant can have different therapeutic properties and potencies.
- **Sustainable Supply Chain:** Ethical suppliers should be able to provide detailed information about where and how their herbs are sourced, ensuring that they are collected in a way that protects both the plant populations and the surrounding ecosystem. Suppliers should also be aware of and comply with local regulations, including obtaining proper permits for wild harvesting. Additionally, it's important to verify that no endangered species are being sourced and that efforts are made to give back to the communities involved in harvesting, ensuring fair compensation and support for traditional knowledge (*Sustainable Herbs Initiative*, n.d.).
- **Testing and Quality Control:** Reputable suppliers often conduct tests for contaminants like heavy metals, pesticides, and microorganisms. They should be willing to provide certificates of analysis upon request.
- **Latin Names:** Ensure the herbs are labeled with their full Latin names. Common names can vary regionally and may refer to different plants in different areas.

- **Harvest Date and Shelf Life:** Look for herbs with a recent harvest date. Most dried herbs maintain their potency for about a year if stored properly.
- **Reputation and Transparency:** Choose suppliers with good reputations in the herbal community. They should be transparent about their sourcing and quality control practices.

By keeping these factors in mind when purchasing herbs, you ensure that you're getting the highest quality materials for your herbal practice. Remember, each of these criteria contributes to the overall quality and efficacy of the herbs you'll be using in your remedies.

Sourcing high-quality herbs from reputable suppliers is a skill that develops over time. By consistently applying these criteria in your purchasing decisions, you'll not only ensure the quality of your herbal preparations but also contribute to the overall integrity of the herbal industry. Remember, every purchase you make is a vote for the kind of practices you want to see in the world of herbal medicine. Choose wisely, and your herbal practice will thrive as a result.

Building Relationships with Suppliers

In the world of herbal sourcing, knowledge is power, but relationships are key. Building strong connections with reputable suppliers can provide you with a consistent source of high-quality herbs and invaluable insights into the world of herbal production. This section explores strategies for cultivating these important relationships.

Here are key ways to build and maintain relationships with herb suppliers:

- **Ask Questions:** Don't hesitate to inquire about sourcing, quality control, and sustainability practices.
- **Provide Feedback:** Let suppliers know about the quality of their products, both positive and negative.

- **Attend Herbal Events:** Conferences, workshops, and herb walks are great places to meet ethical suppliers.
- **Support Local:** When possible, support local herb farms and wildcrafters. This allows for greater transparency and reduces transportation impacts.
- **Join Herbal Organizations:** Many herbal associations provide resources for finding reputable suppliers.

These relationships are a two-way street. As you learn from suppliers, your feedback and support will help shape a more transparent and sustainable herbal industry. A network of connections becomes an invaluable resource in your herbal journey, providing you with access to high-quality herbs, expert knowledge, and a community of like-minded practitioners. You can visit the Resources section for a list of suppliers.

Wildcrafting: Harvesting Herbs from the Wild

Wildcrafting, the practice of harvesting plants from their natural habitat, offers a profound connection to the natural world and can provide herbs

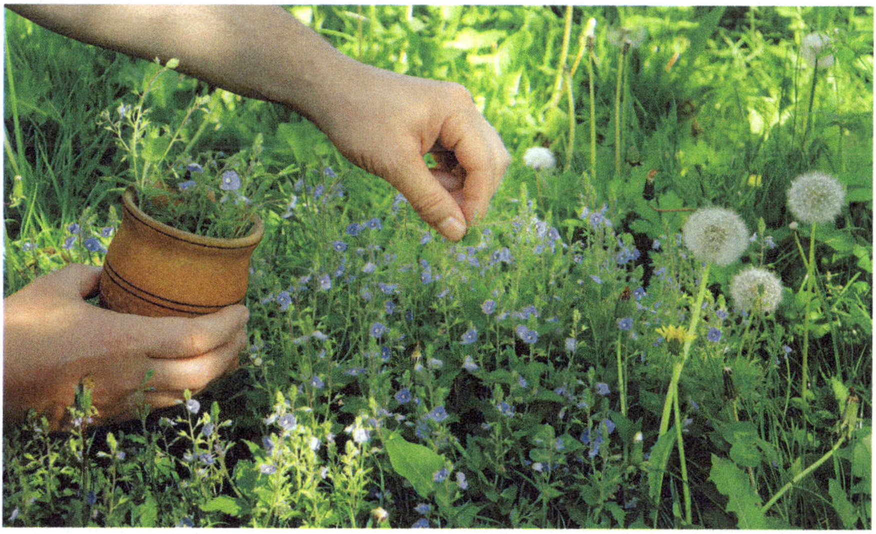

of unparalleled freshness and potency. However, this practice comes with significant responsibilities and requires a deep understanding of both plants and ecosystems. In this section, we'll explore the essentials of ethical wildcrafting, from plant identification to sustainable harvesting practices.

Cultivate When Possible

Growing your own herbs ensures a sustainable supply and allows you to control quality from seed to harvest. Sustainable cultivation practices, including organic growing methods, help reduce the environmental impact of herb production and ensure that the soil and surrounding ecosystems remain healthy (*Sustainable Herbs Initiative*, n.d.).

Plant Identification in the Wild

When foraging, accurate plant identification becomes even more critical than when purchasing herbs. The stakes are higher, as misidentification can lead to harvesting the wrong plant, potentially endangering your health or damaging fragile ecosystems. Here are key considerations for plant identification in the wild:

- **Know Your Ecosystem:** Understand the typical plants in your area, including any endangered or protected species.
- **Consider Look-alikes:** Be aware of any poisonous plants that resemble the herb you're seeking.
- **Observe Habitat:** Note the conditions where the plant is growing. This can aid in identifying the plant and prevent you from harvesting from potentially herbicide-contaminated areas like roadsides.
- **Use Multiple Characteristics:** Don't rely on just one feature for identification. Consider the plant's overall growth habit, leaf arrangement, flower structure, and other unique characteristics.
- **When in Doubt, Don't Harvest:** If you're not 100% certain of a plant's identity, do not collect it.

By adhering to these principles, you significantly reduce the risk of misidentification and ensure that your wildcrafting practices are safe and responsible.

Permission and Access

Familiarize yourself with local laws regarding plant collection, especially on public lands, protected areas, or state-owned territories. Harvesting without permission or knowledge of local regulations can disrupt ecosystems and lead to legal consequences.

Be aware of the cultural significance of plants to Indigenous communities. Respecting Indigenous knowledge and asking permission from tribal governments before accessing sovereign tribal lands for wildcrafting is a crucial part of ethical herbal sourcing.

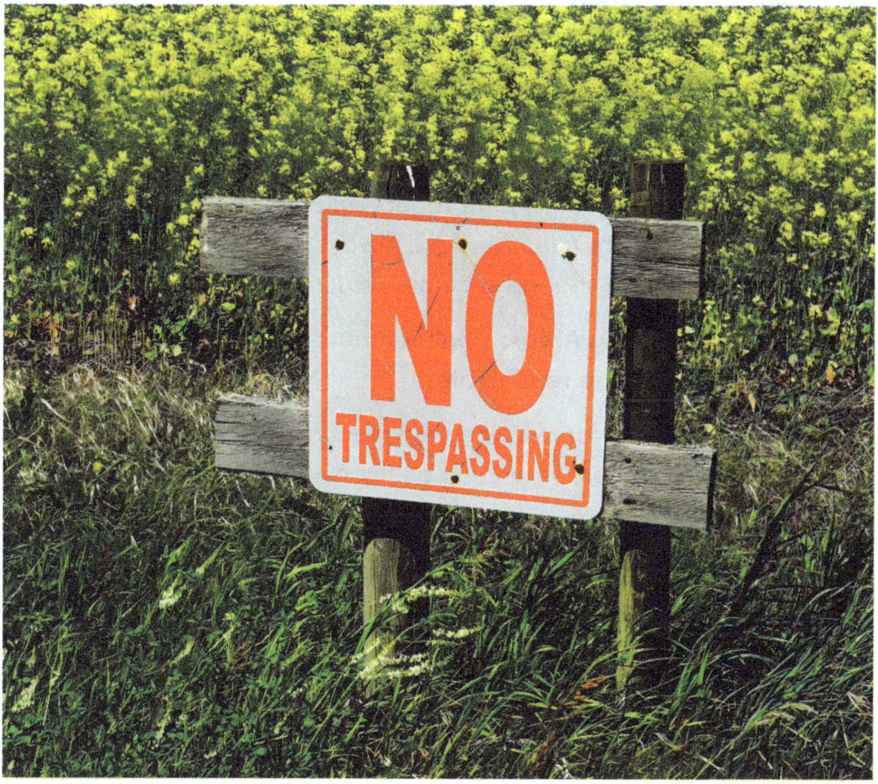

Sustainable Harvesting Practices

Ethical wildcrafting means harvesting in a way that allows plant populations to thrive. The goal is to collect what you need while ensuring the continued health and propagation of the plant species. Here are guidelines for sustainable harvesting:

1. **The 1 in 20 Rule:** Only harvest if there are at least 20 plants for every one you plan to take.
2. **Harvest No More Than 1/3:** Never take more than one-third of a plant or one-third of a stand of plants.
3. **Leave No Trace:** Minimize your impact on the surrounding ecosystem. Don't trample other plants or disturb wildlife.
4. **Use the Right Tools:** Bring clean, sharp tools to make clean cuts that will heal quickly.
5. **Focus on Abundant Species:** Prioritize common plants over rare ones. Many common "weeds" have potent medicinal properties and are abundant in most ecosystems. Common plants like Dandelion are easy to harvest and sustainable. However, it's crucial to refrain from overharvesting even common plants and to harvest them in a manner that promotes the regeneration of the plant population (*Sustainable Herbs Initiative*, n.d.). Always research the conservation status of plants in your area before wildcrafting.
6. **Rotate Harvesting Areas:** Don't return to the same spot year after year. Allow areas to regenerate.
7. **Timing Matters:** Harvest when the plant part you need is at its peak potency. This varies depending on the herb and the part used.
8. **Never Harvest Bark from Live Trees:** Harvesting bark can severely damage or kill a tree. Only collect bark from fallen branches or with explicit permission in managed forest areas.

By following these practices, you ensure that your harvesting activities contribute to, rather than detract from, the health of wild plant populations.

Avoiding Contaminated Areas

When wildcrafting, it's crucial to be aware of potential sources of contamination that could affect the quality and safety of the herbs you harvest. Here are key areas to avoid:

- **Avoid Roadsides:** Plants near roads can accumulate pollutants from vehicle exhaust and, more importantly, are often sprayed with herbicides.
- **Steer Clear of Agricultural Areas:** These may be contaminated with pesticides or herbicides.
- **Be Wary of Water Sources:** Be cautious when harvesting plants near water sources, especially stagnant water or areas prone to flooding. While water is essential for plant growth, certain conditions may increase the risk of contamination.
- **Check for Industrial Activity:** Avoid areas near factories, mines, or other industrial sites that might contaminate soil or water.

By being mindful of these potential sources of contamination, you ensure that the herbs you harvest are not only potent but also free from harmful pollutants.

Processing and Storing Wildcrafted Herbs

Proper handling of wildcrafted herbs is crucial to preserving their quality. The care you take in processing and storing your harvest can significantly impact the potency and shelf life of your herbs. Follow these guidelines:

1. **Clean Carefully:** Gently remove any dirt, insects, or unwanted plant parts by rinsing in water before hanging to dry.
2. **Dry Promptly:** Begin the drying process as soon as possible after harvesting. Use a well-ventilated, shady area or a dehydrator set to a low temperature.

3. **Store Properly:** Once completely dry, store herbs in airtight containers away from light and heat.
4. **Label Thoroughly:** Include the plant's name, date and location of harvest, and any other relevant information.

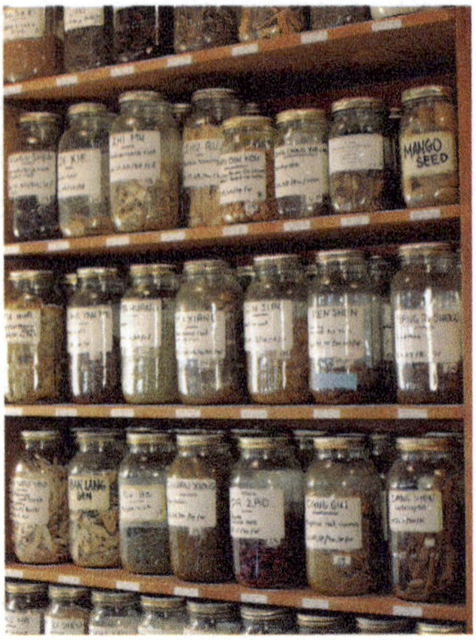

By following these processing and storage practices, you ensure that your wildcrafted herbs retain their potency and remain safe for use.

Ethical wildcrafting is as much about what you leave behind as what you take. By following these guidelines, you not only ensure the quality of your herbs but also contribute to the health and sustainability of wild plant populations. Remember, as a wildcrafter, you are a steward of the natural world, and your practices can have a lasting impact on the ecosystems you interact with.

Final Thoughts on Sourcing

Sourcing high-quality herbs is the cornerstone of effective and ethical herbal practice. By understanding the importance of mastering plant identification skills, knowing what to look for when purchasing, building relationships with suppliers, and practicing ethical wildcrafting, you set the stage for creating potent and safe herbal remedies that not only benefit your personal practice but also contribute to the long-term sustainability of herbal medicine.

CHAPTER 4:
HERB GARDENING FOR BEGINNERS

The art and science of cultivating herbs is a journey that connects you intimately with the plants you'll use in your herbal practice. Whether you have a sprawling backyard or just a sunny windowsill, growing your own herbal medicine can provide you with a sustainable supply of high-quality, fresh plant material for your remedies. This chapter will guide you through the essentials of establishing and maintaining a thriving herb garden, empowering you to take control of the entire process from seed to harvest.

As we explore the world of herb gardening, we'll cover everything from basic plant requirements to troubleshooting common issues. You'll learn how to create the ideal environment for your herbs, choose the right plants for your space and needs, and maintain your garden throughout the seasons. This chapter will give you the skills and confidence to grow medicinal herbs even if you've never gardened.

Understanding Plant Requirements

At the heart of successful herb gardening lies a fundamental understanding of what plants need to thrive. Each plant species has its own preferences, but there are general principles that apply to most herbs. By mastering these basics, you'll create an environment where your herbs can flourish.

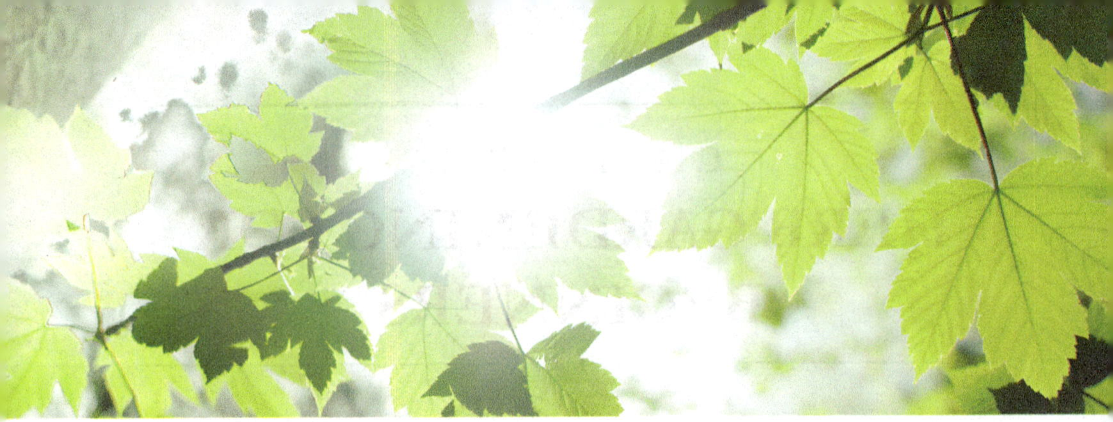

Light: The Energy Source

Light is the primary energy source for plants, driving photosynthesis and influencing growth patterns. When it comes to herbs, light requirements can vary significantly:

- Many culinary and medicinal herbs, such as Basil and Rosemary, thrive in full sun, requiring at least 6 hours of direct sunlight daily.
- Others, like Lemon Balm and Chamomile, can tolerate partial shade, making them more versatile in garden placement.

To manage light effectively:

1. Use a reliable planting guide to determine the specific light requirements for each plant species in your garden.
2. Observe your garden space throughout the day to identify areas of full sun, partial shade, and full shade.
3. Position sun-loving herbs in the brightest spots, while shade-tolerant species can occupy areas that receive less direct light.
4. For indoor gardens, south-facing windows typically provide the most light. If natural light is scarce, think about utilizing grow lights as a supplement.

Remember, too much light can be as problematic as too little. Signs of excessive light exposure include leaf scorching or bleaching. On the other hand, insufficient light often results in leggy, weak growth and pale leaves.

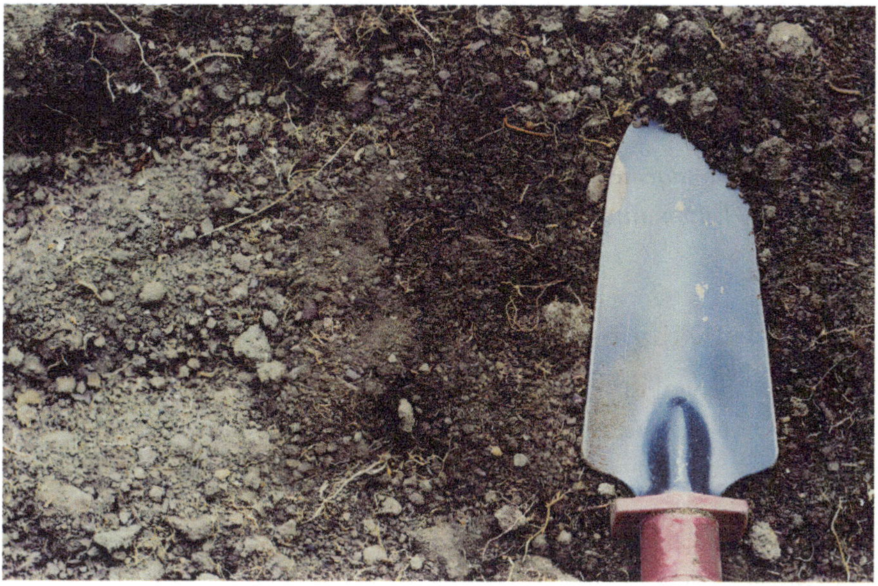

Soil: The Foundation of Health

The soil is more than just a medium for holding plants; it's a complex ecosystem that provides nutrients, water, and oxygen to plant roots. Creating the right soil environment is crucial for herb health:

- Most herbs prefer well-draining, fertile soil with a pH between 6.0 and 7.0.
- Soil texture affects drainage and nutrient retention. A loamy soil, which is a balanced mix of sand, silt, and clay, is ideal for most herbs.

To optimize your soil:

1. Test your soil pH using a home test kit or ask your local agricultural extension service.
2. Amend acidic soils with lime to raise pH, or add sulfur to lower pH in alkaline soils.
3. Improve soil structure and fertility by incorporating organic matter such as compost or well-rotted manure.

4. Use a high-quality potting mix specifically for herbs and vegetables for container gardening.

Proper soil management is an ongoing process. Regular addition of organic matter will help maintain soil health and structure over time.

Water: Finding the Right Balance

Water is essential for plant life, but finding the right balance is key. Too much water can lead to root rot, while too little causes drought stress. Here's how to get it right:

- Most herbs prefer soil that is kept consistently moist, but not waterlogged.
- Watering deeply and less frequently encourages deeper root growth, making plants more resilient to drought.

Watering tips:

1. Water early in the morning to reduce evaporation and allow leaves to dry before nightfall, minimizing disease risk.
2. Use your finger to check soil moisture before watering. If the top inch of soil feels dry, it's time to water.
3. Consider using a drip irrigation system or soaker hose for efficient, targeted watering.
4. For potted herbs, ensure containers have adequate drainage holes to prevent water accumulation.

Remember, different herbs have different water needs. Mediterranean herbs like Rosemary and Lavender prefer drier conditions, while moisture-loving herbs like Peppermint and Holy Basil require more frequent watering.

Nutrients: Feeding Your Herbs

While herbs are generally less demanding than many other plants, proper nutrition is still important for robust growth and optimal flavor or medicinal potency.

Nutrient management strategies:

1. Before planting, incorporate compost or well-rotted manure into the soil to provide a base level of nutrients.
2. During the growing season, apply a balanced, organic fertilizer according to package instructions, typically every 4–6 weeks.
3. Watch for signs of nutrient deficiencies, such as yellowing leaves (nitrogen deficiency) or purple leaf undersides (phosphorus deficiency).
4. Consider foliar feeding with compost tea or seaweed extract for a quick nutrient boost.

By understanding and meeting these basic plant requirements, you'll create an environment where your herbs can thrive. In the next section, we'll explore how to adapt these principles to different gardening situations and spaces.

Adapting to Your Space and Lifestyle

One of the beauties of herb gardening is its adaptability. Whether you have acres of land or just a kitchen windowsill, there's a way to grow herbs. Let's explore how to tailor your herb garden to your specific circumstances.

Assessing Your Space

The first step in planning your herb garden is to honestly assess the space you have available. This will inform everything from plant selection to gardening methods:

- For those with outdoor space, consider factors like sun exposure, proximity to water sources, and existing landscaping.
- If you're working with an indoor space, evaluate available light, humidity levels, and temperature fluctuations.

Space assessment tips:

1. Create a simple sketch of your available area, noting sunny and shady spots.
2. Consider vertical spaces: walls, fences, and balconies can all be utilized for herb growing.
3. Don't forget about microclimates within your space. Areas near walls or large rocks may offer unique growing conditions.

Time and Commitment

Gardening can be as time-consuming or as low-maintenance as you make it. Be realistic about the time you can dedicate to your herb garden:

- Some herbs, like Rosemary, are relatively low-maintenance once established.
- Others, such as Holy Basil, require more frequent attention for harvesting and preventing bolting.

Time management strategies:

1. Start small. It's better to have a few well-tended herbs than a large, neglected garden.

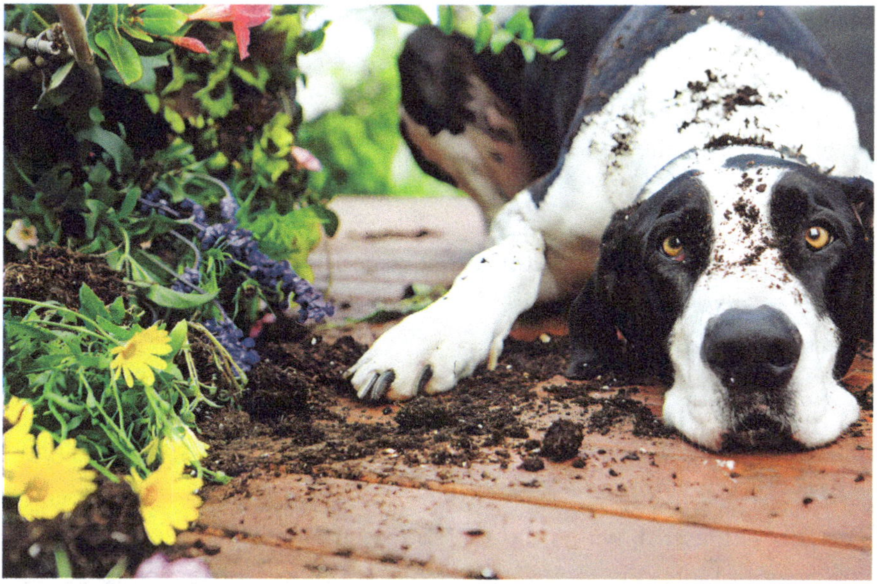

2. Choose herbs that match your availability. If you're often away, focus on drought-tolerant species like Lavender, Rosemary, Echinacea, Calendula, and St. John's Wort.
3. Implement time-saving techniques like mulching to reduce watering and weeding needs.

Pet-Friendly Gardening

Those who have furry friends should prioritize creating a garden that is safe for both plants and pets:

- Some common herbs, like Aloe Vera, can be toxic to cats and dogs.
- Others, like Valerian, may be irresistible to cats and need protection.

Pet-safe gardening tips:

1. Research each herb's potential effects on pets before planting.

2. Consider creating physical barriers around your herb garden to prevent pet access.
3. Grow pet-friendly herbs like Rosemary, which is safe if ingested in small quantities.

By tailoring your herb garden to your specific space and lifestyle, you'll create a sustainable practice that brings joy and abundance without overwhelming you.

Outdoor Herb Gardening

For those blessed with outdoor space, the possibilities for growing medicinal plants are vast. Let's explore various approaches to outdoor herb cultivation.

Integrating Herbs into Your Landscape

Herbs can be both beautiful and functional additions to your existing landscape:

- Many herbs, like Lavender, have attractive foliage and flowers that can enhance your garden's aesthetic.
- Integrating herbs into your landscape can create a cohesive, edible garden design.

Landscape integration tips:

1. Use herbs as border plants along pathways or to define garden areas.
2. Incorporate herbs into rock gardens for a Mediterranean-inspired look.

3. Plant low-growing Chamomile or Peppermint between steppingstones to create a fragrant, whimsical pathway in your herb garden.

Raised Bed Herb Gardens

Raised beds offer numerous advantages for herb growing:

- They provide excellent drainage and allow for better soil control.
- Raised beds warm up earlier in spring, extending the growing season.

Creating raised bed herb gardens:

1. Choose a sunny location with good air circulation.
2. Build beds no wider than 4 feet to allow easy access from all sides.
3. Fill with a high-quality soil mix enriched with compost.
4. Group herbs with similar water and light requirements together.

Vertical Herb Gardens

Vertical gardening is an excellent solution for maximizing space:

- It allows you to grow more herbs in a smaller footprint.
- Vertical gardens can create stunning visual displays.

Vertical gardening techniques:

1. Use hanging baskets for trailing herbs like Peppermint and Lemon Balm.
2. Create a herb wall using a palette or specialized vertical planter, incorporating a variety of herbs such as Lavender, Rosemary, and Chamomile.
3. Utilize trellises or supports for climbing herbs like Passionflower.

Container Herb Gardens

Container gardening offers flexibility and can be adapted to various outdoor spaces:

- It's ideal for patios, balconies, or areas with poor soil.
- Containers allow you to easily move herbs to optimize growing conditions.

Container herb gardening tips:

1. Choose containers with adequate drainage holes.
2. Use a high-quality potting mix specifically formulated for containers.
3. Group containers with similar water needs for efficient irrigation.
4. Consider self-watering containers for low-maintenance herb growing.

By exploring these outdoor gardening options, you can create a herb garden that not only meets your needs for fresh herbs but also enhances the beauty of your outdoor space.

Indoor Herb Gardening

Don't let the lack of outdoor space deter you from herb gardening. Many herbs thrive indoors, providing year-round access to fresh plants.

Windowsill Herb Gardens

Windowsills are often the go-to spot for indoor herbs:

- South-facing windows typically provide the most light, ideal for sun-loving herbs.
- East or west-facing windows can work well for herbs that tolerate partial shade.

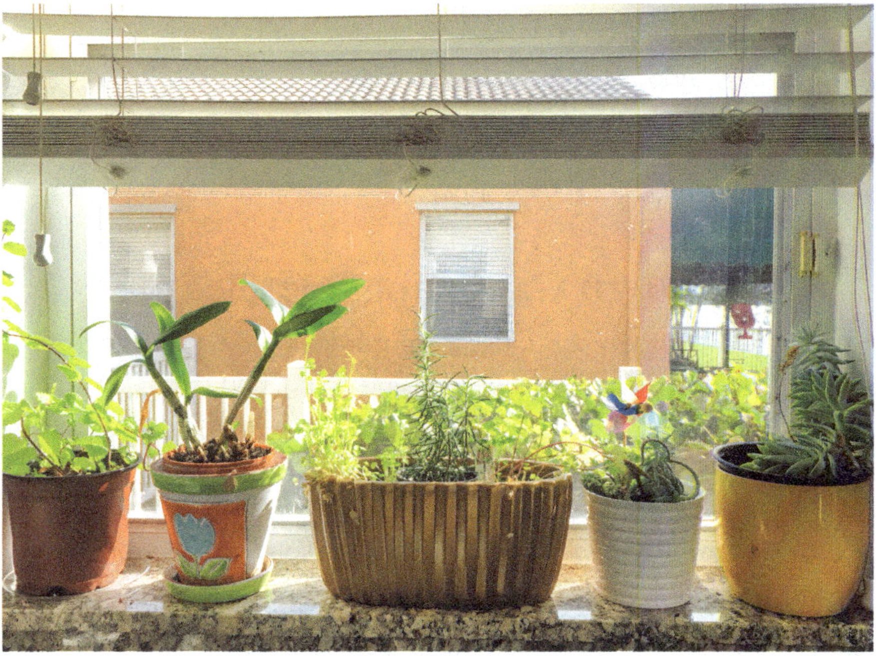

Windowsill gardening tips:

1. Choose compact herb varieties suited for container growing, such as Peppermint, Chamomile, Lavender, and Rosemary.
2. Rotate plants regularly to ensure even growth and prevent leaning.
3. Use saucers under pots to protect windowsills from water damage.

Indoor Vertical Gardens

Vertical gardening isn't just for outdoors—it can be adapted for indoor use too:

- Wall-mounted herb gardens can be both functional and decorative.
- Vertical gardens make efficient use of limited indoor space.

Indoor vertical gardening ideas:

1. Install an indoor-use living wall system.
2. Create a tiered plant stand to maximize vertical space.
3. Use over-the-door shoe organizers as pocket planters for herbs.

Essential Herb Gardening Supplies

Having the right tools can make herb gardening more enjoyable and efficient. Here's a list of essential herb gardening tools:

- **Gloves:** Choose comfortable, water-resistant gloves that allow dexterity.
- **Hand trowel:** Essential for planting, transplanting, and working soil.
- **Pruning shears:** For harvesting herbs and maintaining plant shape.
- **Watering can or hose with adjustable nozzle:** For precise watering.
- **Plant labels:** To keep track of different herb varieties.
- **Potting soil and containers:** For container gardening.
- **Compost bin:** To create your own nutrient-rich soil amendment.
- **pH testing kit:** To monitor soil acidity levels.

Invest in quality tools that will last, and always clean and store them properly after use.

Planting Your Herb Garden

With your space prepared and supplies at hand, it's time to start planting. Whether you're starting from seeds, seedlings, or cuttings, proper planting techniques are crucial for success.

Starting From Seeds

Growing herbs from seeds is economical and allows you to choose from a wider variety of plants:

- Certain herbs, like Chamomile and Fennel, grow quickly from seed.
- Certain plants, like Rosemary and Lavender, are better suited for planting small seedlings.

Seed starting tips:

1. Use a sterile seed-starting mix to prevent disease.
2. Plant seeds at the depth recommended on the packet.
3. Keep soil consistently moist but not waterlogged.
4. Provide bottom heat for faster germination.
5. Once seedlings develop true leaves, transplant them to larger containers or the garden.

Planting Seedlings

Purchasing seedlings gives you a head start and can be a good option for slower-growing herbs:

- Choose healthy seedlings with no signs of disease or pest damage.
- Avoid rootbound plants, which may struggle to establish in the garden.

Transplanting tips:

1. Harden off indoor-grown seedlings before planting outdoors.
2. Dig a hole slightly larger than the root ball.
3. Gently loosen the roots if they're tightly bound.
4. Plant at the same depth as the seedling was growing in its container.
5. Water thoroughly after planting.

Propagating From Cuttings

Many herbs can be propagated from cuttings, allowing you to multiply your plants for free:

- Soft-stemmed herbs, like Peppermint and Lemon Balm, root easily in water.
- Woody herbs like Rosemary and Lavender can be propagated in soil.

Propagation steps:

1. Take 4–6-inch cuttings from healthy, non-flowering stems.
2. Remove lower leaves, leaving 2–3 sets at the top.
3. For soft-stemmed herbs, place in water and change the water every few days.
4. For woody herbs, dip the cut end in rooting hormone and plant in moist potting mix.
5. Keep cuttings in a warm, bright spot out of direct sunlight until roots develop.

By mastering these planting techniques, you'll be able to start and expand your herb garden with confidence.

Maintaining Your Herb Garden

A thriving herb garden requires ongoing care and attention. Regular maintenance not only keeps your plants healthy but also helps you address issues early.

Watering

Proper watering is crucial for herb health:

- Most herbs prefer soil that's allowed to dry slightly between waterings.
- Water deeply and less frequently to encourage deep root growth.

Watering best practices:

1. Water at the base of plants to keep foliage dry and prevent fungal diseases.
2. Water in the morning to reduce evaporation and allow leaves to dry before nightfall.
3. Use mulch to retain soil moisture and reduce watering frequency.

Fertilizing

While herbs generally don't require heavy feeding, some nutritional support can boost growth:

- Overfertilizing can lead to reduced flavor and medicinal potency.
- Organic, slow-release fertilizers are ideal for herbs.

Fertilizing tips:

1. Apply a balanced, organic fertilizer in spring when growth resumes.
2. Side-dress heavy feeders like Holy Basil and Peppermint with compost mid-season.
3. Avoid fertilizing late in the season to prevent tender new growth before winter.

Pruning and Harvesting

Regular pruning and harvesting promote bushy growth and prevent herbs from becoming woody:

- Many herbs can be harvested continuously throughout the growing season.
- Proper pruning techniques vary depending on the herb species.

Pruning and harvesting guidelines:

1. Never remove more than one-third of the plant at one time.
2. Pinch back the growing tips of herbs like Peppermint and Holy Basil to encourage branching.
3. Harvest herbs in the morning after the dew has dried but before the heat of the day sets in for the best flavor and medicinal potency.
4. Use sharp, clean tools to make clean cuts and prevent disease transmission.
5. For leafy herbs, harvest the oldest leaves first, allowing new growth to continue.

Pest and Disease Management

Even well-maintained gardens can face pest and disease issues. The key is early detection and intervention:

- Many common garden pests, like aphids and spider mites, can affect herbs.
- Fungal diseases, particularly in humid conditions, can be problematic for some herbs.

Organic pest and disease control strategies:

1. Inspect plants regularly for signs of pests or disease.
2. Encourage beneficial insects by planting flowers like Marigolds and Alyssum nearby.
3. Use organic insecticidal soaps or neem oil for pest infestations.
4. Improve air circulation to prevent fungal diseases.

5. Remove and dispose of severely affected plants to prevent spread.

If you need further assistance with pest and disease management in your herb garden, consider reaching out to your local agricultural extension office. These offices, often affiliated with state universities, provide a wealth of resources and expertise for gardeners and farmers. They can help with identifying specific pests or diseases affecting your herbs and provide tailored advice for your local growing conditions.

Other helpful resources include:

- **Master gardener programs:** These programs, also often affiliated with local extension offices, consist of trained volunteers who can offer gardening advice and troubleshooting.
- **Local gardening clubs or organizations:** Connecting with other herb gardeners in your area can provide a great opportunity to share knowledge and learn from others' experiences.
- **Online gardening forums and communities:** Many online platforms host active communities of gardeners where you can ask questions, share photos, and get advice from experienced growers.

While pest and disease issues can be frustrating, they are a normal part of gardening. With careful observation, proactive management, and the right resources, you can keep your herb garden healthy and thriving.

Seasonal Care

Your herb garden's needs will change with the seasons. Adapting your care routine accordingly will ensure year-round success. Table 1 outlines essential gardening tasks for each season to maintain a healthy and productive herb garden.

Table 1: Seasonal Care Guide for Herb Gardens

Season	Gardening Tasks
Spring	• Prune back any winter damage. • Fertilize perennial herbs as new growth emerges. • Sow seeds or plant seedlings after the last frost.
Summer	• Water more frequently during hot, dry periods. • Harvest regularly to encourage continued growth. • Mulch to retain moisture and suppress weeds.
Fall	• Reduce watering as temperatures cool. • Harvest herbs for drying or freezing before the first frost. • Plant Garlic and other fall-planted herbs.
Winter	• Protect tender perennial herbs with mulch or row covers. • Bring potted herbs indoors or to a sheltered location. • Continue to grow cold-hardy herbs.

By following these maintenance practices, you'll create a healthy, productive herb garden that provides a bountiful harvest throughout the growing season.

Harvesting and Preserving Herbs

The ultimate reward of herb gardening is the harvest. Knowing when and how to harvest, as well as how to preserve your bounty, will ensure you can enjoy your herbs year-round.

Timing Your Harvest

The timing of your harvest can significantly affect the flavor and potency of your herbs:

- Harvest most leafy herbs in the morning after the dew dries but before peak heat.
- Harvest flowering herbs just before the flowers open for maximum essential oil content.

Proper Harvesting Techniques

How you harvest can impact both the quality of your harvest and the health of your plants:

- Use clean, sharp tools to make clean cuts and prevent disease transmission.
- Never harvest more than one-third of a plant at a time to ensure continued growth.

Harvesting best practices:

1. For leafy herbs, cut stems just above a leaf intersection to promote branching.
2. Harvest root herbs at the end of the growing season, when the plant has stored maximum energy.
3. Collect seeds when they're fully ripe, but before they scatter.

Drying Herbs

Drying is one of the oldest and most effective methods of preserving herbs:

- Air drying works well for herbs with low moisture content, like Rosemary and Lavender.
- Herbs with higher moisture content may require a dehydrator to prevent mold.

Drying methods:

1. Air drying: Tie herbs in small bundles and hang in a warm, dry, well-ventilated area.
2. Oven drying: Spread herbs on a baking sheet and dry at the lowest temperature setting.
3. Dehydrator: Follow the manufacturer's instructions for temperature and time.

Freezing Herbs

Freezing can preserve the fresh flavor of herbs, especially those with high water content:

- Herbs like Lemon Balm, Peppermint, and Holy Basil can be effectively preserved through freezing.
- Frozen herbs retain many of their medicinal properties and are best used in preparations like teas or tinctures rather than as fresh remedies. When using frozen herbs, allow them to thaw completely before incorporating them into your herbal preparations.

Freezing techniques:

1. Ice cube method: Chop herbs, place in ice cube trays, cover with water or oil, and freeze.
2. Flat freeze method: Lay herb leaves flat on a baking sheet, freeze, then transfer to a storage container.

Troubleshooting Common Issues

Even experienced gardeners encounter problems from time to time. Knowing how to identify and address common plant issues will help you maintain a healthy herb garden. If you're unsure about a problem or need expert advice, don't hesitate to seek help. Your local nursery or agricultural extension office can be a valuable resource. Many of these offices accept plant samples for diagnosis—simply place a sample of the affected plant in a sealed plastic bag and bring it in for examination.

Table 2 presents common plant symptoms, their potential causes, and practical solutions to help you diagnose and address issues in your herb garden. Use this table as a quick reference guide when troubleshooting problems with your plants.

Proper care and regular monitoring can prevent many gardening problems. Don't be discouraged if you encounter issues—each challenge is an opportunity to learn and become a better gardener. For more in-depth troubleshooting guidance, refer to the **Resources** section at the back of this book, which lists reputable websites, books, and local organizations that can provide expert advice on herb gardening challenges.

Table 2: Troubleshooting Guide for Common Herb Garden Problems

Plant Symptom	Causes	Solutions
Yellowing Leaves	Poor soil health, nutrient deficiencies, overwatering or underwatering	Improve soil with compost, test soil for nutrient balance, adjust watering schedule to avoid stress
Wilting Plants	Overwatering, underwatering, or poor drainage	Ensure proper drainage, water deeply and less frequently, adjust watering to the plant's needs
Pest Infestations	Weak or stressed plants, lack of biodiversity, improper spacing, weeds	Strengthen plants by improving soil and water management, practice companion planting, weed control.
Fungal Diseases	High humidity, poor airflow, overcrowding, overwatering	Space plants properly, water early in the day, avoid overhead watering
Poor Growth	Nutrient deficiencies, poor soil, lack of sunlight, pest damage	Add compost or organic matter, test soil for nutrients, ensure proper sunlight, control pests early

Embracing the Herb Gardening Journey

Herb gardening is a journey of continuous learning and discovery, where each success and challenge contributes to your growing expertise. By understanding basic plant requirements, troubleshooting common issues, and experimenting with new herbs and techniques, you can create and maintain a thriving medicinal herb garden that not only provides powerful ingredients for your herbal remedies but also offers a meditative practice and a way to connect with nature.

CHAPTER 5:
PREPARATION METHODS

The journey from raw herbs to effective remedies is a transformative process that combines ancient wisdom with modern understanding. This chapter will guide you through the art and science of preparing three fundamental types of herbal remedies: teas, herbal tinctures, and salves. By mastering these methods, you'll be able to harness the healing power of plants in ways that are both potent and practical for everyday use.

Whether you're steeping a soothing cup of Chamomile tea, crafting a potent Echinacea tincture, or creating a healing Calendula salve, the principles and techniques you'll learn here will form the foundation of your herbal practice.

Essential Tools and Equipment

Before we dive into the preparation methods, let's ensure you have the right tools at your disposal. Having the proper equipment not only makes the process easier, but also helps ensure the quality and safety of your herbal preparations.

Here's a list of essential tools for making teas, herbal tinctures, and salves:

- **Mason jars:** For storing tinctures and infused oils
- **Wire mesh strainers:** For separating plant material from liquid
- **Cheesecloth:** For finer straining of tinctures and oils
- **Measuring cups and spoons:** For accurate ingredient measurements
- **Funnels:** For transferring liquids without spills
- **Glass bottles:** For storing finished tinctures

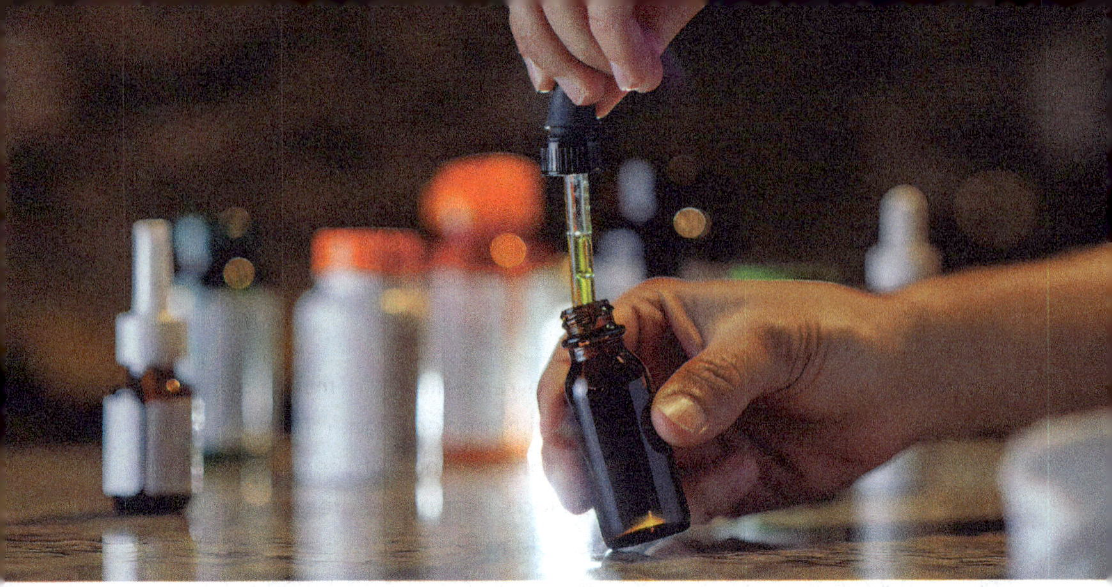

- **Labels:** For marking your preparations with content and date
- **Blender or food processor:** For grinding herbs (optional)
- **Double boiler:** For making salves
- **Small glass jars or tins:** For storing salves

Always remember to thoroughly clean and sterilize all tools before use. This prevents contamination and ensures the purity of your herbal preparations. You can sterilize glass and metal tools by boiling them for 10 minutes or running them through a dishwasher's hot cycle.

Ingredients

The ingredients you use in your herbal preparations are just as important as the herbs themselves. Here are the key ingredients you'll need for each of the three preparation methods we're focusing on:

1. Teas
    - Purified or spring water
    - Honey or other natural sweeteners (optional)

2. Tinctures
   - High-proof alcohol (vodka or grain alcohol, at least 80 proof)
   - Glycerin (for alcohol-free tinctures)
3. Salves
   - Carrier oil (such as olive oil, coconut oil, or almond oil)
   - Beeswax

Each of these ingredients plays a specific role in the preparation process:

- Water in teas acts as a solvent, extracting water-soluble compounds from the herbs.
- Alcohol in tinctures extracts both water-soluble and alcohol-soluble compounds, resulting in a more potent preparation.
- Oils in salves extract fat-soluble compounds and provide a base for topical application.
- Beeswax in salves gives the preparation its solid consistency.
- Glycerin extracts water-soluble compounds and serves as a sweet, alcohol-free preservative suitable for children and those avoiding alcohol.

Always opt for high-quality ingredients. The purity of your base ingredients will directly impact the quality of your final product.

Appropriate Dosage

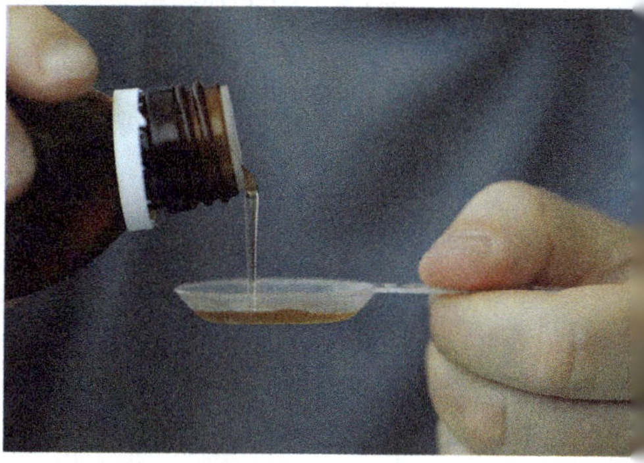

Determining the correct dosage for herbal remedies is a crucial aspect of safe and effective use. Unlike standardized pharmaceutical drugs, herbal preparations can vary in potency based on factors such as growing conditions, harvest time, and preparation method. Therefore, it's essential to approach dosing with care and knowledge.

It's crucial to consult reliable sources when determining dosages. Reputable herbals, pharmacopoeias, and plant monographs provide valuable information on appropriate dosing for specific herbs. Some useful resources include:

- The Herbal Academy's Herbal Dosage Calculator
- Mountain Rose Herbs' Dosage Guidelines
- American Herbal Pharmacopoeia monographs

Remember, while these tools and resources are helpful, they don't replace professional medical advice. Always consult with a qualified healthcare provider, especially if you have pre-existing health conditions or are taking other medications.

Factors influencing dosage include:

1. The specific herb and its potency.
2. The form of preparation (tea, tincture, or salve).
3. Individual factors such as age, weight, and overall health.
4. The condition is being addressed.
5. Potential interactions with other medications or supplements.

When determining dosage, consider the following guidelines:

- **Teas:** Start with 1 teaspoon of dried herb per cup of water, steeped for 5–10 minutes. Drink 1–3 cups daily, unless otherwise indicated for specific herbs.
- **Tinctures:** Begin with a low dose, typically 20–30 drops (1–1.5 ml) taken 2–3 times daily. Adjust as needed based on effects and tolerability.
- **Salves:** Apply a thin layer to the affected area 2–3 times daily, or as needed.

Always start with the lowest recommended dose and gradually increase if necessary. Pay attention to how your body responds and adjust accordingly (Bone & Mills, 2013).

Storage

Proper storage is crucial for maintaining the potency and safety of your herbal preparations. Each type of preparation has specific storage requirements:

1. Teas
   - Store dried herbs in airtight containers away from light and heat.
   - Keep prepared teas refrigerated and use within 24–48 hours.
2. Tinctures
   - Store in dark glass bottles to protect from light.
   - Keep in a cool, dark place. Properly stored tinctures can last for years.
3. Salves
   - Store in airtight glass jars or tins.
   - Keep in a cool, dark place. Most salves will last 6–12 months.

General Storage Tips:

- Label all preparations with the contents, date of preparation, and expiration date.
- Use clean, dry utensils when handling preparations to prevent contamination.
- Check stored preparations regularly for signs of spoilage such as mold, off odors, or changes in color or consistency.

By following these storage guidelines, you'll ensure that your herbal remedies remain potent and safe for use when you need them.

Safety Precautions

While herbal remedies can be powerful healing tools, it's important to approach their use with respect and caution. Here are some key safety considerations:

- **Allergies:** Before using any new herb, do a patch test to check for allergic reactions.
- **Interactions:** Some herbs can interact with medications or other supplements. Always research potential interactions and consult with a healthcare provider if you're taking medications.
- **Contraindications:** Certain herbs may not be suitable for people with specific health conditions or during pregnancy and breastfeeding. Always check contraindications before use.
- **Quality:** Use high-quality, properly identified herbs from reputable sources to avoid contamination or misidentification.
- **Moderation:** Even beneficial herbs can have side effects if used excessively. Follow recommended dosages and use periods.

Remember, natural doesn't always mean safe for everyone. It's crucial to approach herbal medicine with knowledge and respect for its potency (Ekor, 2013; Bone & Mills, 2013).

Documentation and Record-Keeping

Keeping detailed records of your herbal preparations and their effects is an invaluable practice. It helps you understand what does and does not work for your body so you can make adjustments, if necessary. Here's what you should include in your herbal journal:

1. Herb information: Name, source, date of purchase or harvest
2. Preparation details: Method, ingredients, and date prepared

3. Dosage used
4. Intended use
5. Observed effects (both positive and negative)
6. Any modifications to the preparation or dosage.

This documentation will not only help you refine your herbal practice but also provide valuable information to share with healthcare providers if needed.

Preparation Types

Now, let's delve into the specific methods for preparing teas, herbal tinctures, and salves. Each method extracts and preserves herbal constituents in different ways, making them suitable for various applications.

Water-Based Preparations: *Herbal Teas*

Herbal teas, also known as infusions, are one of the simplest and most accessible forms of herbal medicine. They're excellent for extracting water-soluble compounds from herbs.

Instructions:

1. Use 1 teaspoon of dried herb (or 1 tablespoon of fresh herb) per cup of water.
2. Bring water to a boil, then remove from heat.
3. Add the herbs to a tea infuser or directly into the water.
4. Cover and steep for 5–10 minutes (or longer for roots and bark).
5. Strain and enjoy.

Suggested Herbs:

- ✓ Ashwagandha
- ✓ Chamomile
- ✓ Dandelion
- ✓ Elderberry
- ✓ Fennel
- ✓ Ginger
- ✓ Holy Basil
- ✓ Hops
- ✓ Lavender
- ✓ Lemon Balm
- ✓ Licorice
- ✓ Nettle
- ✓ Passionflower
- ✓ Peppermint
- ✓ Rhodiola

Precautions: *Some herbs may have stimulant effects or interact with medications. Always check for potential contraindications before using new herbs as teas.*

Alcohol-Based Preparations: *Herbal Tinctures*

Herbal tinctures are concentrated liquid extracts that use alcohol as a solvent. The body easily absorbs them; they are potent, and they have a long shelf life.

Some may wonder, *Why alcohol? Why not glycerin?* Alcohol is a more potent solvent compared to glycerin, meaning it can extract a wider range of plant compounds, including both water-soluble and alcohol-soluble constituents. Herbs containing alkaloids, resins, and other compounds, which are difficult to extract in water or glycerin, greatly benefit from this.

Alcohol also has better preservative properties than glycerin, ensuring a longer shelf life for the tincture. Alcohol-based tinctures can last for several years when stored properly, while glycerites have a shorter shelf life, typically around 1–2 years.

With this in mind, glycerin is a good choice for herbs that are high in mucilage, such as Marshmallow root, or for those who prefer to avoid alcohol for personal or health reasons. Glycerin is sweeter than alcohol, making the tincture more suitable for children.

Instructions:

1. Fill a clean glass jar 1/3 to 1/2 full with dried herbs.
2. Cover completely with alcohol (vodka or grain alcohol, at least 80 proof).
3. Seal the jar and store in a cool, dark place for 4–6 weeks, shaking daily.
4. Strain through cheesecloth, squeezing out all liquid.
5. Store the tincture in dark glass bottles.

Suggested Herbs:

- ✓ Ashwagandha
- ✓ Astragalus
- ✓ Burdock
- ✓ Calendula
- ✓ Dandelion
- ✓ Echinacea
- ✓ Elderberry
- ✓ Goldenseal
- ✓ Hops
- ✓ Lavender
- ✓ Licorice
- ✓ Rhodiola
- ✓ St. John's Wort
- ✓ Turmeric
- ✓ Valerian

Best for Glycerin-Based Tinctures:

- ✓ Aloe Vera
- ✓ Chamomile
- ✓ Fennel
- ✓ Holy Basil
- ✓ Lemon Balm
- ✓ Licorice
- ✓ Nettle
- ✓ Passionflower

- ✓ Peppermint
- ✓ Rosemary

Can be used with either Alcohol or Glycerin:

- ✓ Elderberry
- ✓ Ginger

Precautions: *Alcohol-based tinctures may not be suitable for everyone. Always start with a low dose and be aware of potential interactions with medications.*

Oil-Based Preparations: *Salves*

Salves are semi-solid preparations used topically. They are highly effective in delivering herbs directly to the skin, resulting in targeted effects.

Instructions:

1. Infuse herbs in oil (1:5 ratio of herb to oil) over low heat for 2–3 hours.
2. Strain the oil through cheesecloth.
3. Add 1 oz of beeswax per 1 cup of infused oil.
4. Heat gently until the beeswax melts, then pour into containers to cool.

Suggested Herbs:

- ✓ Aloe Vera
- ✓ Calendula
- ✓ Ginger
- ✓ Lavender
- ✓ Peppermint
- ✓ Rosemary
- ✓ St. John's Wort
- ✓ Turmeric

Precautions: *Always do a patch test before applying a new salve to larger areas of skin. Some individuals may be sensitive to certain herbs or carrier oils.*

Other Preparation Types

While this book focuses on teas, herbal tinctures, and salves, it's worth noting that there are many other ways to prepare and use herbs. These include capsules, juices, creams, steam inhalations, baths, and mouthwashes. Each type of preparation has its own benefits and applications.

As you grow more comfortable with these basic preparations, you may wish to explore other methods. Always approach new preparation techniques with the same care and attention to safety that we've discussed in this chapter.

Preparation Is Key

Preparing your own herbal remedies is a rewarding and empowering practice. By mastering the techniques for making teas, tinctures, and salves, you're taking a significant step towards natural wellness. Remember, the key to successful herbal preparations lies in using quality ingredients, following proper techniques, and always prioritizing safety. Keep learning, keep experimenting, and enjoy the process of becoming your own herbalist.

CHAPTER 6:
HERBAL REMEDIES AND RECIPES

Welcome to the heart of our herbal journey. In this chapter, we'll provide a wide array of herbal remedy recipes using herbs that are designed to support the body and provide a variety of health benefits. Each section focuses on a particular body part, providing you with practical, easy-to-follow recipes for teas, tinctures, and salves.

As you explore these remedies, remember that herbal medicine is both an art and a science. While we provide specific recipes and dosages, it's important to listen to your body and adjust as needed. Everyone's body is unique, and what works perfectly for one person may need tweaking for another.

Important note: Before we delve into the remedies, it's important to note that while these herbal preparations can be powerful allies in supporting various therapeutic actions, they should not replace professional medical advice.

In this chapter, we'll cover a range of therapeutic applications and the systems supported by our herbal allies, including:

1. Immune System Support
2. Cognitive Function and Memory Support
3. Detoxification, Cleanse, and Urinary Tract Support
4. Digestive System Support
5. Energy and Vitality Enhancement
6. Pain Management and Inflammation

7. Skin, Hair, and Beauty
8. Sleep Support and Relaxation
9. Stress and Anxiety Reduction
10. Women's Health

We'll provide multiple herbal remedies, explaining the specific properties of each herb and how they work synergistically in the preparations to support the corresponding body part or system. We'll also include tips on when and how to use each remedy, as well as any precautions you should be aware of. Remember, you can always review the details of each herb by referring to **Appendix I: Plant Monographs** at the end of the book.

Immune System Support

Staying healthy and fighting off seasonal illnesses can be a challenge, but nature provides us with potent herbs to support our immune system. This collection of remedies taps into the power of time-honored herbs to bolster your body's natural defenses.

Echinacea and Elderberry Immune Boost Tincture

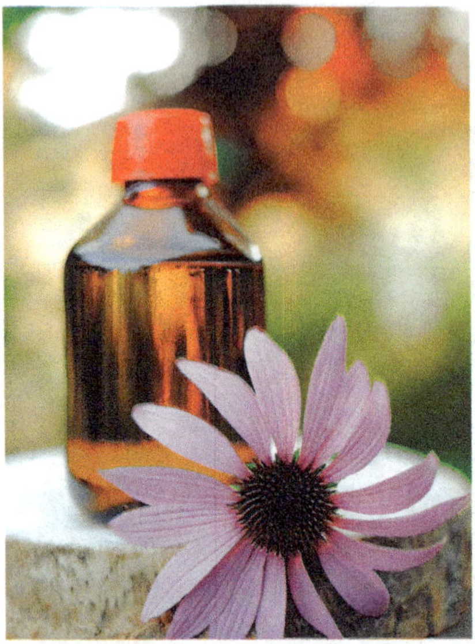

Echinacea is known to stimulate the production of white blood cells, particularly natural killer cells, which are crucial in fighting off viral infections. It also contains compounds that may help reduce inflammation and combat bacterial infections.

Elderberry, on the other hand, has shown impressive antiviral properties, particularly against influenza viruses. Studies have found that elderberry can shorten the duration of flu symptoms and reduce their severity. It's rich in antioxidants and vitamin C, which further support immune function.

Ingredients:

- 2 parts dried Echinacea root
- 1 part dried Elderberries
- 80-proof vodka or brandy

Instructions:

1. Fill a clean glass jar 1/3 full with the herbs.
2. Pour alcohol over the herbs until completely covered.
3. Seal the jar and store in a cool, dark place for 4–6 weeks, shaking daily.
4. Strain through cheesecloth and store in a dark glass bottle.

Usage: Take 1/4 to 1/2 teaspoon up to 3 times daily at the first sign of illness. For prevention during cold and flu season, take once daily.

Note: Do not use Echinacea continuously for more than 8 weeks. Take a 1–2 week break before resuming use. Those with autoimmune conditions should consult a healthcare provider before using Echinacea.

Source: Tiralongo et al., 2016

Ginger and Holy Basil Tea for Chest Colds

Ginger possesses warming properties that aid in clearing congestion and has demonstrated antiviral effects against respiratory syncytial virus, a common culprit in respiratory infections. It also has anti-inflammatory properties that can help soothe a sore throat (Chan et al., 2010)

Holy Basil is considered an adaptogen, helping the body cope with stress, which can weaken the immune system. It also has expectorant properties—helping to clear mucus from the lungs—and has shown antibacterial effects against strains that commonly cause respiratory infections.

Ingredients:

- 1 tsp fresh grated Ginger
- 1 tsp dried Holy Basil leaves
- 1 cup hot water
- Honey to taste (optional)

Instructions:

1. Place Ginger and Holy Basil in a tea infuser or bag.
2. Pour hot water over the herbs and steep for 10 minutes.
3. Remove herbs, add honey if desired, and drink while warm.

Usage: Drink 2–3 cups daily during a chest cold. For prevention, enjoy a cup daily during cold and flu season.

Source: Ryan et al., 2011

Calendula and Goldenseal Antimicrobial Tincture

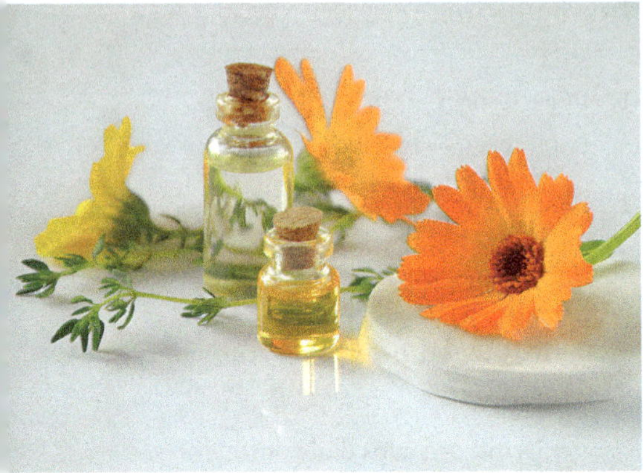

Calendula: Known for its antimicrobial and anti-inflammatory properties, Calendula helps fight off infections and soothe inflammation.

Goldenseal: Contains berberine, a potent antibacterial compound that is effective against oral and general infections.

Ingredients:

- 2 parts dried Calendula flowers
- 1 part dried Goldenseal root
- 80-proof vodka or brandy (for extraction)

Instructions:

1. Place the dried Calendula and Goldenseal into a clean glass jar, filling it about 1/3 full with the herbs.
2. Pour the vodka (or brandy) over the herbs, ensuring they are completely submerged.
3. Seal the jar tightly and store it in a cool, dark place for 4–6 weeks. Shake the jar daily to ensure the herbs are well-extracted.
4. After the infusion period, strain the tincture through cheesecloth or a fine mesh sieve, and transfer the liquid into a dark glass bottle with a dropper.

Usage: For antimicrobial support, take 1/4 to 1/2 teaspoon up to three times daily. This can be used for minor infections, to support immune function, or as part of your oral hygiene routine.

Source: Bone & Mills, 2013

Astragalus and Echinacea Immune-Boosting Tincture

Astragalus: Supports and strengthens the immune system, helping the body fight off infections.

Echinacea: Stimulates the immune system and has antiviral and antibacterial properties.

Ingredients:

- 2 parts dried Astragalus root
- 1 part dried Echinacea root
- 80-proof vodka or brandy

Instructions:

1. Fill a clean glass jar 1/3 full with the herbs.
2. Pour alcohol over the herbs until completely covered.
3. Seal the jar and store in a cool, dark place for 4–6 weeks, shaking daily.
4. Strain through cheesecloth and store in a dark glass bottle.

Usage: Take 1/4 to 1/2 teaspoon up to 3 times daily during cold and flu season.

Source: Bone & Mills, 2013

Astragalus and Elderberry Immune Tea

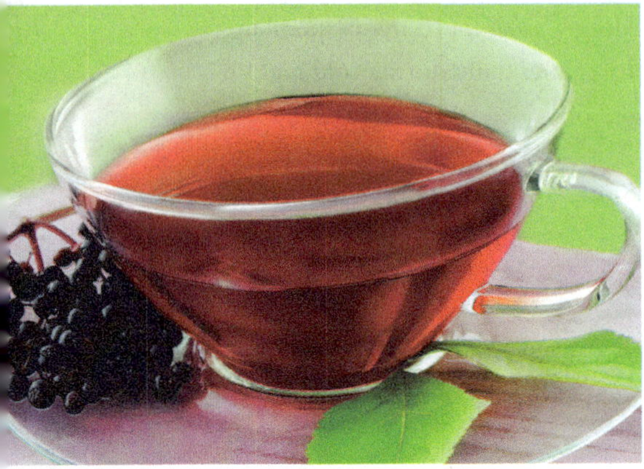

Astragalus: Supports immune function by boosting the body's resistance to infections and acting as an adaptogen to reduce stress on the immune system.

Elderberry: Known for its antiviral properties, particularly effective against cold and flu viruses, and rich in antioxidants and vitamin C.

Ingredients:

- 1 tsp dried Astragalus root
- 1 tsp dried Elderberries
- 1 cup hot water

Instructions:

1. Combine the Astragalus and Elderberries in a tea infuser or directly into a cup.
2. Pour hot water over the herbs and steep for 10–15 minutes.
3. Strain the herbs or remove the infuser, and drink while warm.

Usage: Drink 1–2 cups daily to support immune function, especially during cold and flu season.

Source: Ulbricht et al., 2014

Cognitive Function and Memory Support

Sharpening your mental edge and enhancing cognitive function can be a game-changer in both your personal and professional life. Explore this array of herbal remedies designed to support brain health, focus, and relaxation.

Rosemary and Holy Basil Memory Enhancing Tincture

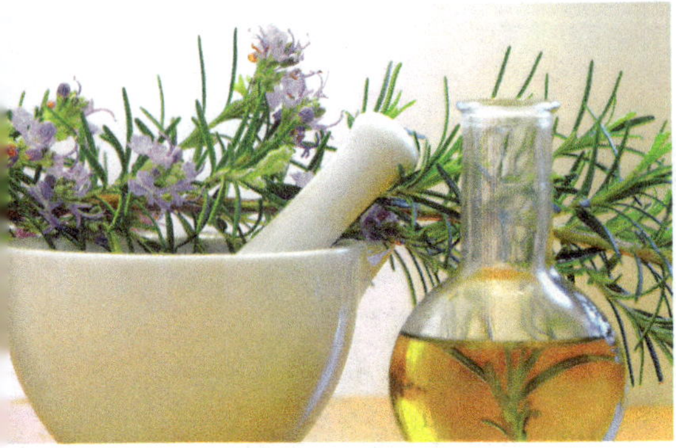

Rosemary: Traditionally used to enhance memory and increase circulation to the brain.

Holy Basil: Known as an adaptogen, it helps reduce stress while improving cognitive function.

Ingredients:

- 2 parts dried Rosemary leaves
- 1 part dried Holy Basil leaves
- 80-proof vodka or brandy

Instructions:

1. Place the dried Rosemary and Holy Basil into a clean glass jar, filling it about 1/3 full with the herbs.
2. Pour vodka or brandy over the herbs, ensuring they are fully submerged.
3. Seal the jar and store in a cool, dark place for 4–6 weeks, shaking daily.
4. After the infusion period, strain the liquid through cheesecloth into a dark glass bottle with a dropper.

Usage: Take 1/4 to 1/2 teaspoon twice daily to support memory and cognitive function.

Source: Bone & Mills, 2013

Rosemary and Peppermint Focus Tea

Rosemary: Supports memory and mental clarity.

Peppermint: Improves alertness and concentration, while also being calming to the nervous system.

Ingredients:

- 1 tsp dried Rosemary leaves
- 1 tsp dried Peppermint leaves
- 1 cup hot water
- Honey to taste (optional)

Instructions:

1. Place Rosemary and Peppermint into a tea infuser or directly into a mug.
2. Pour hot water over the herbs and steep for 5–10 minutes.
3. Remove the herbs or infuser and add honey if desired.

Usage: Drink 1–2 cups daily to enhance focus and support cognitive function.

Source: Bone & Mills, 2013

Lemon Balm and Ashwagandha Brain Tincture

Lemon Balm: Promotes calmness and mental clarity, supporting brain function.

Ashwagandha: Reduces stress and improves cognitive function, making it an excellent adaptogen for brain health.

Ingredients:

- 2 parts dried Lemon Balm leaves
- 1 part dried Ashwagandha root
- 80-proof vodka or brandy

Instructions:

1. Place the Lemon Balm and Ashwagandha into a clean glass jar, filling it about 1/3 full with the herbs.
2. Pour vodka or brandy over the herbs, ensuring they are completely submerged.
3. Seal the jar and store in a cool, dark place for 4–6 weeks, shaking daily.
4. Strain the tincture through cheesecloth into a dark glass bottle.

Usage: Take 1/4 to 1/2 teaspoon twice daily to support brain health, focus, and stress reduction.

Source: Cohen et al., 1964

Lemon Balm and Rhodiola Focus-Enhancing Tea

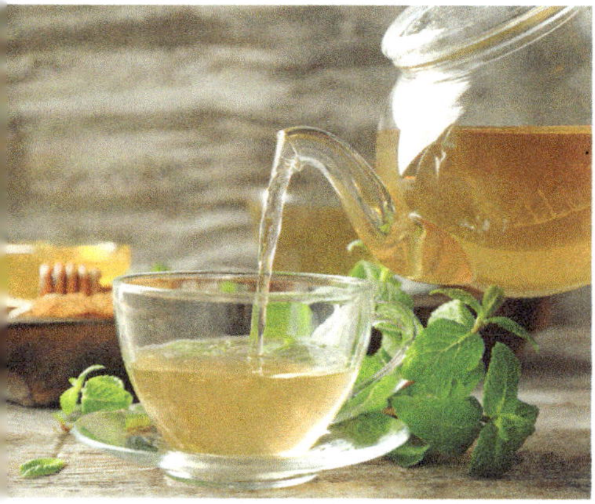

Lemon Balm has been shown to have calming effects while also improving cognitive performance. It may help reduce stress and anxiety, which can interfere with memory and focus.

Rhodiola is an adaptogenic herb that can help the body cope with stress. It's also been shown to reduce mental fatigue and improve performance on cognitive tasks, particularly in stressful situations.

Ingredients:

- 1 tsp dried Lemon Balm leaves
- 1 tsp dried Rhodiola root
- 1 cup hot water
- Honey to taste (optional)

Instructions:

1. Combine Lemon Balm and Rhodiola in a tea infuser or bag.
2. Pour hot water over the herbs and steep for 5–10 minutes.
3. Remove herbs, add honey if desired, and drink.

Usage: Drink 1 cup daily, preferably in the morning or early afternoon, to support focus, and reduce stress.

Note: Rhodiola can have a stimulating effect and may interfere with sleep if taken late in the day. Those with bipolar disorder should avoid Rhodiola, as it may trigger manic episodes.

Source: Ishaque et al., 2012

Peppermint and Lemon Balm Focus Tincture

Peppermint: Enhances alertness and mental clarity while also calming the nervous system.

Lemon Balm: Reduces stress and promotes calmness while supporting cognitive function and focus.

Ingredients:

- 2 parts dried Peppermint leaves
- 1 part dried Lemon Balm leaves
- 80-proof vodka or brandy

Instructions:

1. Place the dried Peppermint and Lemon Balm into a clean glass jar, filling it about 1/3 full with the herbs.
2. Pour vodka or brandy over the herbs, ensuring they are fully submerged.
3. Seal the jar and store in a cool, dark place for 4–6 weeks, shaking daily.
4. Strain the liquid through cheesecloth into a dark glass bottle with a dropper.

Usage: Take 1/4 to 1/2 teaspoon up to 2 times daily to support focus and cognitive function while reducing stress.

Source: Cohen et al., 1964

Detoxification, Cleanse, and Urinary Tract Support

Detoxification and cleansing are crucial for supporting the body's ability to eliminate toxins and maintain optimal organ function. Herbal remedies in this category promote liver and kidney health, help cleanse the urinary tract, and support overall detox processes, ensuring the body stays balanced and healthy.

Burdock and Dandelion Cleansing Tea

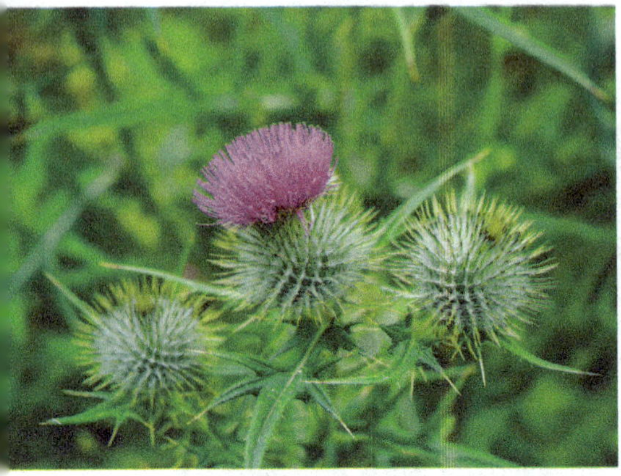

Burdock: Supports detoxification and reduces inflammation.

Dandelion: Acts as a stronger diuretic, promoting bile production and flushing the kidneys.

Supports: Liver and kidney detoxification, stronger diuretic action.

Ingredients:

- 1 tsp dried Burdock root
- 1 tsp dried Dandelion root
- 1 cup hot water

Instructions:

1. Place the Burdock root and Dandelion root in a tea infuser or directly in a cup.
2. Pour hot water over the herbs and steep for 10–15 minutes.
3. Strain the herbs or remove the infuser and drink warm.
4. Optionally, add honey or lemon for taste.

Usage: Drink 1–2 cups daily to promote liver and kidney detox, and to support urinary tract health.

Source: Chan et al., 2010

Turmeric and Ginger Detox Tea

Turmeric is a powerful anti-inflammatory and antioxidant herb. Studies have shown that curcumin, its active compound, supports liver function and may help protect against liver damage. Turmeric also supports the body's natural detoxification processes.

Ginger stimulates digestion and supports liver function. It has antioxidant properties and may help reduce inflammation in the body. Ginger also supports healthy circulation, which is important for overall detoxification.

Ingredients:

- 1 tsp dried Turmeric root
- 1 tsp dried Ginger root
- 1/8 tsp Black Pepper (to enhance turmeric absorption)
- 1 cup hot water
- Honey to taste (optional)
- Lemon slice (optional)

Instructions:

1. Place Turmeric, Ginger, and Black Pepper in a tea infuser or bag.
2. Pour hot water over the herbs and steep for 10–15 minutes.
3. Remove herbs, add honey and lemon slice if desired, and drink while warm.

Usage: Drink 1 cup daily, preferably in the morning, to support detoxification.

Note: Turmeric may interact with blood thinners and may lower blood sugar. Those with gallbladder issues should consult a healthcare provider before using Turmeric in medicinal doses.

Source: Hewlings & Kalman, 2017

Burdock and Nettle Detox Tea

Burdock: Helps eliminate toxins, supports kidney function, and reduces inflammation.

Nettle: Acts as a mild diuretic while providing essential nutrients like iron and calcium.

Supports: Urinary tract health, kidney function, nutrient replenishment.

Ingredients:

- 1 tsp dried Burdock root
- 1 tsp dried Nettle leaf
- 1 cup hot water

Instructions:

1. Place the Burdock root and Nettle leaf in a tea infuser or directly in a cup.
2. Pour hot water over the herbs and let them steep for 10–15 minutes.
3. Strain the herbs or remove the infuser and drink warm.
4. Optionally, add honey for taste.

Usage: Drink 2–3 cups daily to gently support urinary tract health, detoxification, and nutrient replenishment.

Source: Chan et al., 2010

Astragalus and Dandelion Detox Tea

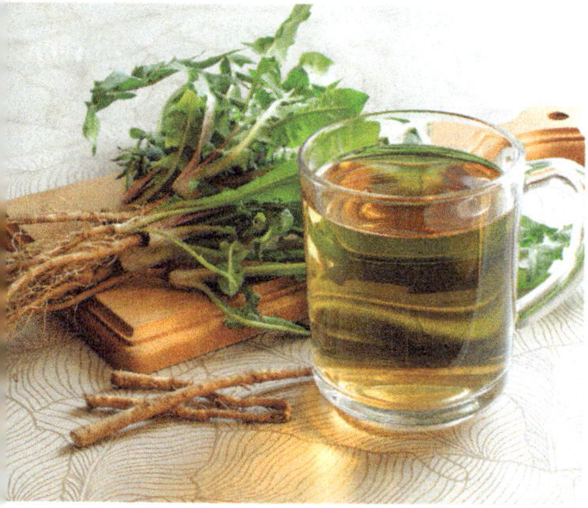

Astragalus: Supports the body's natural detoxification processes and helps protect the liver.

Dandelion: Stimulates bile production, aids in digestion, and supports liver and kidney function.

Ingredients:

- 1 tsp dried Astragalus root
- 1 tsp dried Dandelion root
- 1 cup hot water

Instructions:

1. Place the Astragalus and Dandelion in a tea infuser or directly into a cup.
2. Pour hot water over the herbs and steep for 10–15 minutes.
3. Strain the herbs or remove the infuser and drink warm.

Usage: Drink 1–2 cups daily to support detoxification and kidney health.

Source: Bone & Mills, 2013

Astragalus and Nettle Kidney Support Tincture

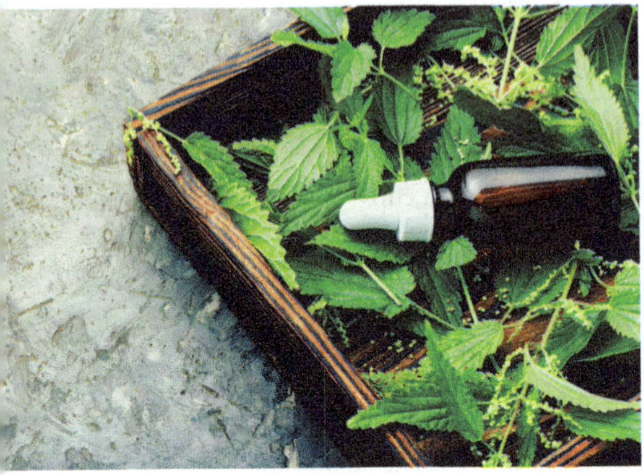

Astragalus: Helps support kidney health and enhances the body's ability to eliminate toxins.

Nettle: Acts as a mild diuretic, supporting urinary tract health and providing essential nutrients like iron and calcium.

Ingredients:

- 2 parts dried Astragalus root
- 1 part dried Nettle leaf
- 80-proof vodka or brandy

Instructions:

1. Place the dried Astragalus root and Nettle leaves into a clean glass jar, filling it about 1/3 full with the herbs.
2. Pour vodka or brandy over the herbs, ensuring they are fully submerged.
3. Seal the jar and store in a cool, dark place for 4–6 weeks, shaking daily.
4. Strain the tincture through cheesecloth into a dark glass bottle with a dropper.

Usage: Take 1/4 to 1/2 teaspoon 1–2 times daily to support kidney function and detoxification.

Source: Bone & Mills, 2013

Digestive System Support

Cultivating a healthy and resilient digestive system is the foundation for overall well-being. This collection of herbal remedies offers a natural approach to supporting various aspects of digestive function, from occasional discomfort to enhanced nutrient absorption.

Peppermint and Fennel Digestive Ease Tincture

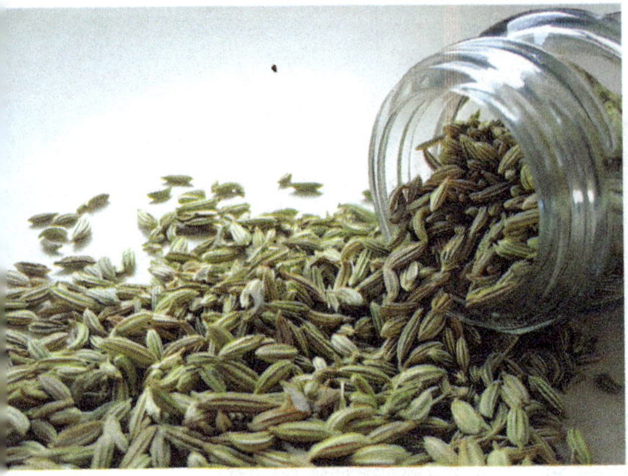

Peppermint is well-known for its digestive benefits. It can help relieve indigestion, reduce bloating, and ease nausea. Peppermint has antispasmodic properties that can help relieve digestive cramps and spasms.

Fennel is a carminative herb, meaning it helps prevent and expel gas from the digestive tract. It can help relieve bloating, indigestion, and may help stimulate the production of digestive enzymes.

Ingredients:

- 2 parts dried Peppermint leaves
- 1 part Fennel seeds
- 80-proof vodka or brandy

Instructions:

1. Fill a clean glass jar 1/3 full with the herbs.
2. Pour alcohol over the herbs until completely covered.
3. Seal the jar and store in a cool, dark place for 4–6 weeks, shaking daily.
4. Strain through cheesecloth and store in a dark glass bottle.

Usage: Take 1/4 to 1/2 teaspoon before or after meals to aid digestion.

Note: Peppermint may exacerbate acid reflux in some individuals. Those with gallstones should consult a healthcare provider before using Peppermint medicinally.

Source: Khanna et al., 2014

Ginger and Chamomile Soothing Digestive Tea

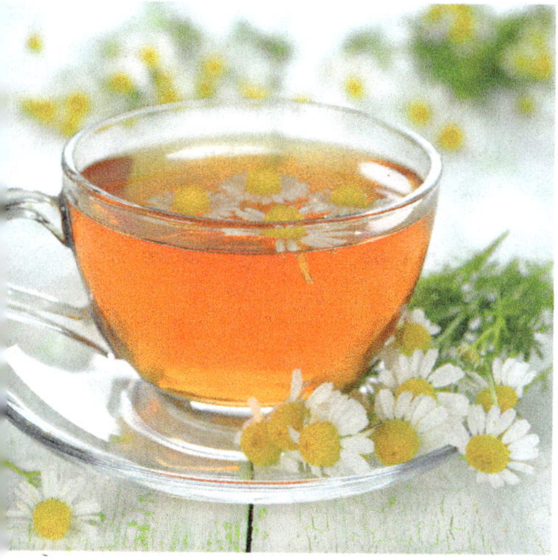

Ginger is a powerful digestive aid. It can help relieve nausea, reduce inflammation in the digestive tract, and may help stimulate the production of digestive enzymes. Ginger has also been shown to help with gastric emptying, which can be beneficial for those with slow digestion.

Chamomile is known for its calming properties, which extend to the digestive system. It can help soothe an upset stomach, reduce inflammation, and may help relieve symptoms of irritable bowel syndrome (IBS).

Ingredients:

- 1 tsp fresh grated Ginger (or 1/2 tsp dried ginger)
- 1 tsp dried Chamomile flowers
- 1 cup hot water
- Honey to taste (optional)

Instructions:

1. Combine Ginger and Chamomile in a tea infuser or bag.
2. Pour hot water over the herbs and steep for 10 minutes.
3. Remove herbs, add honey if desired, and drink.

Usage: Drink 1–2 cups daily to support digestive health, or as needed for digestive discomfort.

Note: Those with ragweed allergies may be sensitive to Chamomile. Ginger may interact with blood thinners and may lower blood sugar.

Source: Ryan et al., 2011

Chamomile and Dandelion Digestive Tea

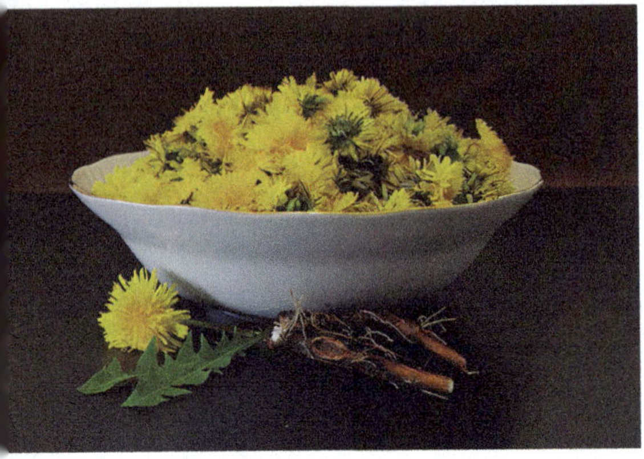

Chamomile: Soothes digestive discomfort and reduces inflammation in the digestive tract.

Dandelion: Supports digestion by stimulating bile production and aiding in the breakdown of fats.

Ingredients:

- 1 tsp dried Chamomile flowers
- 1 tsp dried Dandelion root
- 1 cup hot water
- Honey to taste (optional)

Instructions:

1. Place Chamomile flowers and Dandelion root in a tea infuser or bag.
2. Pour hot water over the herbs.
3. Steep Chamomile for 5 minutes, then remove (to prevent bitter taste).
4. Allow Dandelion root to continue steeping for another 5–10 minutes (10–15 minutes total) to extract its beneficial compounds.
5. Add honey if desired.

Usage: Drink 1 cup 15–30 minutes before meals to support digestion. Can be consumed up to 3 times daily.

Source: Dai et al., 2022

Ginger and Fennel Digestive Tea

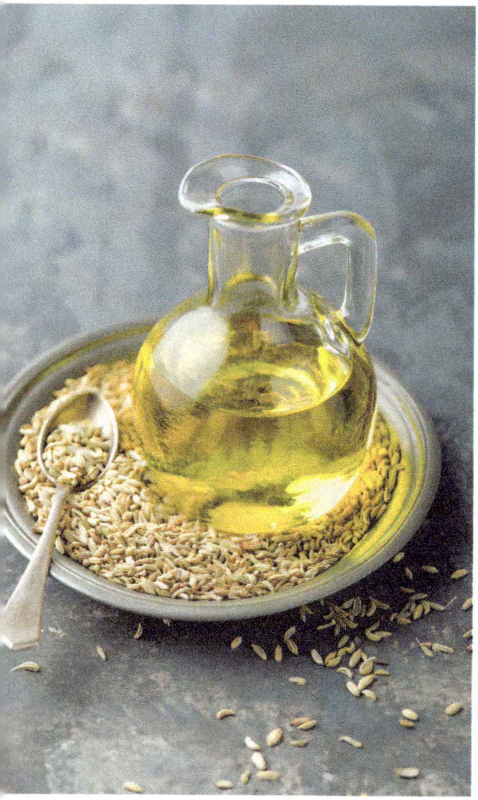

Ingredients:

- 1 tsp dried Ginger root, thinly sliced
- 1 tsp Fennel seeds, lightly crushed
- 1 cup hot water
- Honey (optional)

Instructions:

1. Combine Ginger and Fennel in a tea infuser or bag
2. Pour hot water over herbs
3. Steep covered for 10–15 minutes
4. Strain and add honey if desired

Usage: Drink 1 cup 15–30 minutes before meals to aid digestion and reduce bloating. Can be consumed up to 3 times daily.

Source: Ryan et al., 2011

Ginger: Helps reduce nausea, supports digestion, and relieves inflammation in the digestive tract.

Fennel: A carminative herb that relieves bloating, stimulates digestive enzymes, and reduces gas.

Peppermint and Chamomile Digestive Tea

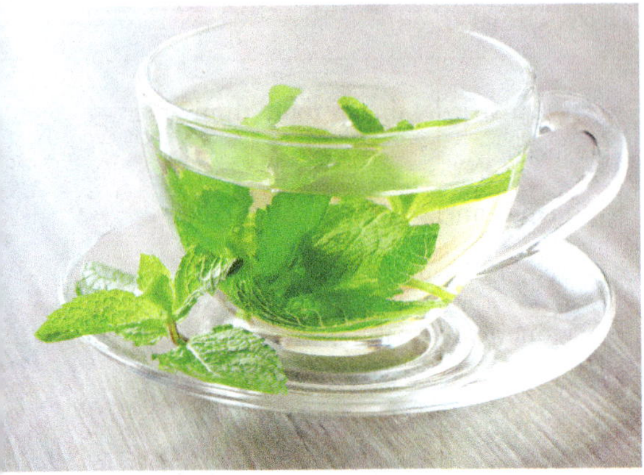

Peppermint: Helps relieve indigestion and bloating, and has antispasmodic properties that soothe digestive discomfort.

Chamomile: Calms and soothes the digestive tract, reducing inflammation and alleviating symptoms of irritable bowel syndrome (IBS).

Ingredients:

- 1 tsp dried Peppermint leaves
- 1 tsp dried Chamomile flowers
- 1 cup hot water

Instructions:

1. Place the Peppermint and Chamomile into a tea infuser or directly into a cup.
2. Pour hot water over the herbs and steep for 10 minutes.
3. Remove the infuser or strain the herbs, and drink warm.

Usage: Drink after meals to relieve indigestion, bloating, and digestive cramps.

Source: Khanna et al., 2014

Energy and Vitality Enhancement

Feeling energized, vibrant, and full of life is essential for living an active, fulfilling existence. Explore this collection of herbal remedies designed to boost your energy levels, support physical and mental endurance, and promote overall vitality.

Ashwagandha and Rhodiola Energy Boost Tea

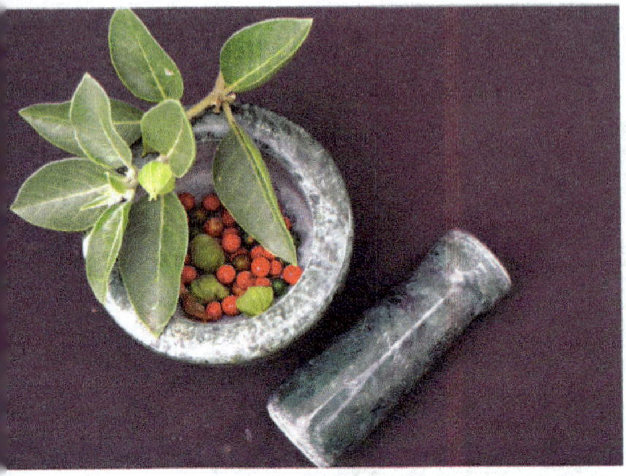

Ashwagandha is a powerful adaptogenic herb that has been used in Ayurvedic medicine for thousands of years. It's known for its ability to enhance energy and reduce fatigue, particularly in the face of chronic stress. Research suggests that Ashwagandha may help improve physical performance and reduce cortisol levels, the body's primary stress hormone.

Rhodiola is another adaptogenic herb that has been shown to combat fatigue and enhance mental performance. It may help increase the body's resistance to various stressors, both physical and mental.

Ingredients:

- 1 tsp dried Ashwagandha root
- 1 tsp dried Rhodiola root
- 1 cup hot water
- Honey to taste (optional)

Instructions:

1. Combine herbs in a tea infuser or bag.
2. Pour hot water over the herbs and steep for 10–15 minutes.
3. Strain and drink.

Usage: Drink 1 cup in the morning to support energy and vitality.

Note: Use Ashwagandha with caution in autoimmune conditions, as it may interact with thyroid medications. Rhodiola can have a stimulating effect and may interfere with sleep if taken late in the day.

Source: Ishaque et al., 2012

Elderberry and Echinacea Immune Support Tea

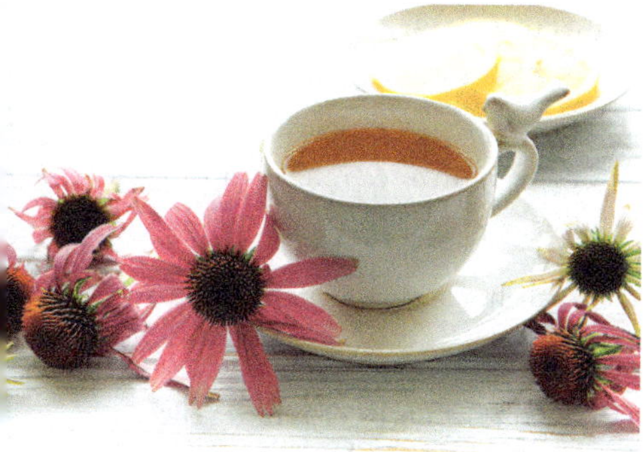

Elderberry: Supports immune function and has traditionally been used during cold and flu season.

Echinacea: Helps stimulate the immune system and may reduce the duration of common colds.

Ingredients:

- 1 tsp dried Elderberries
- 1 tsp dried Echinacea root
- 1/4 tsp dried Ginger root
- 1 cup hot water
- Honey to taste (optional)

Instructions:

1. Combine Elderberries and Echinacea root (and Ginger if using) in a tea infuser or bag.
2. Pour hot water over the herbs.
3. Steep covered for 15 minutes to extract beneficial compounds.
4. Strain herbs and add honey if desired.

Usage: Drink 1 cup up to 3 times daily at the first sign of illness, or 1 cup daily during cold and flu season for immune support.

Note: Not recommended during pregnancy. Those with autoimmune conditions should consult their healthcare provider before using Echinacea.

Source: Ulbricht et al., 2014

Peppermint and Licorice Energy Tea

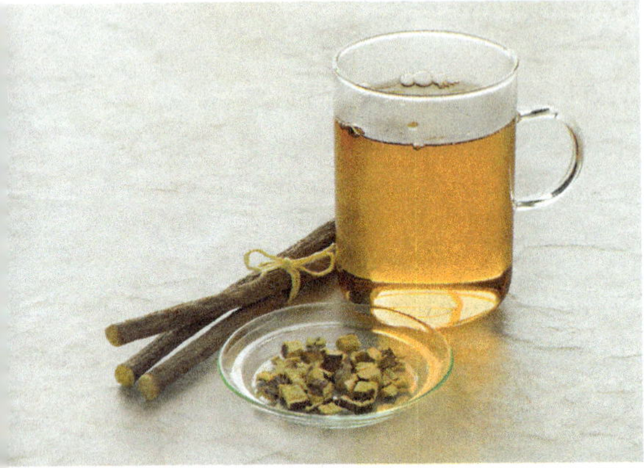

Peppermint: Improves alertness and mental clarity.

Licorice: Supports adrenal health and helps combat fatigue.

Ingredients:

- 1 tsp dried Peppermint leaves
- 1/2 tsp dried Licorice root
- 1 cup hot water
- Honey to taste (optional)

Instructions:

1. Combine the Peppermint and Licorice in a tea infuser or directly in a cup.
2. Pour hot water over the herbs and steep for 5–10 minutes.
3. Strain the herbs or remove the infuser and drink while warm.

Usage: Drink 1 cup in the morning or early afternoon for a gentle energy boost.

Source: Bone & Mills, 2013

Lemon Balm and Rosemary Revitalizing Tea

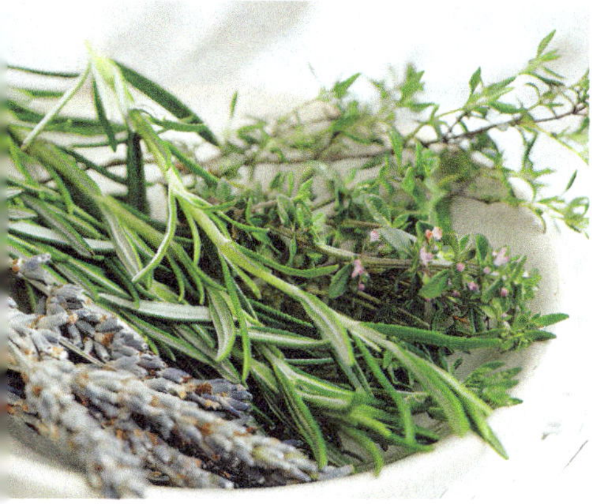

Lemon Balm is known for its calming properties, which support mental clarity.

Rosemary is traditionally used to enhance memory and improve circulation, providing an uplifting effect.

Ingredients:

- 1 tsp dried Lemon Balm leaves
- 1 tsp dried Rosemary leaves
- 1 cup hot water
- Honey to taste (optional)

Instructions:

1. Combine the Lemon Balm and Rosemary in a tea infuser or directly in a cup.
2. Pour hot water over the herbs and steep for 10 minutes.
3. Strain the herbs or remove the infuser and drink warm.

Usage: Drink 1–2 cups daily to support mental clarity and energy.

Source: Cohen et al., 1964

Astragalus and Ashwagandha Energy Tincture

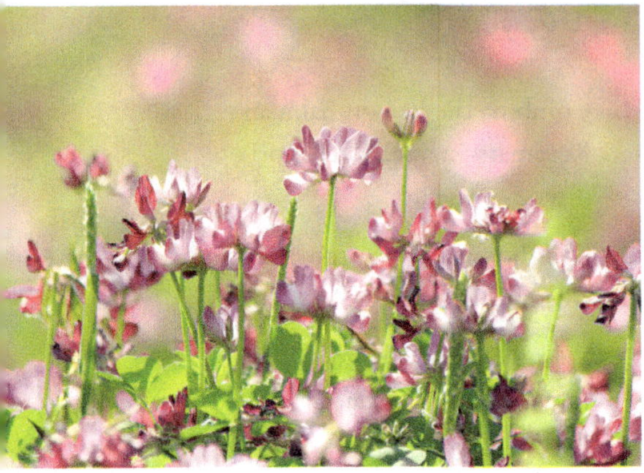

Astragalus: Supports the body's energy production and helps reduce fatigue.

Ashwagandha: An adaptogenic herb that enhances energy, reduces stress, and improves overall vitality.

Ingredients:

- 2 parts dried Astragalus root
- 1 part dried Ashwagandha root
- 80-proof vodka or brandy

Instructions:

1. Fill a clean glass jar 1/3 full with the herbs.
2. Pour alcohol over the herbs until completely covered.
3. Seal the jar and store in a cool, dark place for 4–6 weeks, shaking daily.
4. Strain through cheesecloth and store in a dark glass bottle.

Usage: Take 1/4 to 1/2 teaspoon 1–2 times daily to support energy and vitality.

Source: Bone & Mills, 2013

Pain Management and Inflammation

Discomfort and inflammation can take a toll on our quality of life, but nature offers a wealth of herbal solutions to support the body's natural healing processes. Explore this collection of remedies designed to alleviate pain and reduce inflammation.

Turmeric and Ginger Anti-Inflammatory Tincture

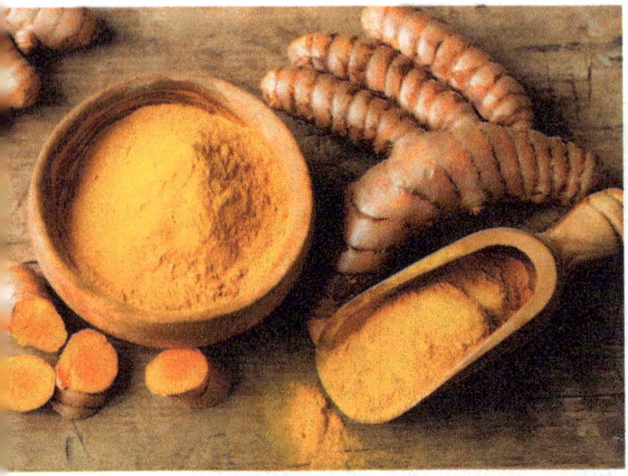

Turmeric contains curcumin, a compound with powerful anti-inflammatory and antioxidant properties. Turmeric is effective in reducing pain and inflammation in conditions such as osteoarthritis and rheumatoid arthritis.

Ginger has been used for centuries to reduce inflammation and relieve pain. It contains compounds called Gingerols that have been shown to have anti-inflammatory and analgesic effects.

Ingredients:

- 2 parts dried Turmeric root
- 1 part dried Ginger root
- 80-proof vodka or brandy
- 1/4 tsp Black Pepper (to enhance Turmeric absorption)

Instructions:

1. Fill a clean glass jar 1/3 full with the herbs.
2. Add Black Pepper.
3. Pour alcohol over the herbs until completely covered.
4. Seal the jar and store in a cool, dark place for 4–6 weeks, shaking daily.
5. Strain through cheesecloth and store in a dark glass bottle.

Usage: Take 1/4 to 1/2 teaspoon 1–3 times daily to reduce inflammation and pain.

Note: Turmeric may interact with blood thinners, which may lower blood sugar. Ginger may also interact with blood thinners, which may lower blood pressure.

Source: Hewlings & Kalman, 2017

Turmeric and Nettle Joint Health Tincture

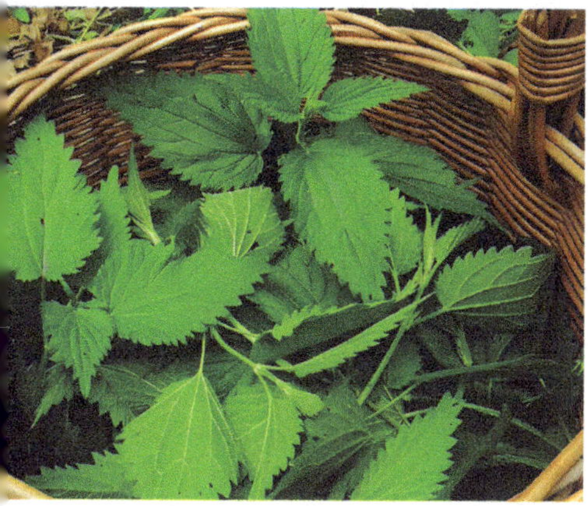

Turmeric: Contains curcumin, a powerful anti-inflammatory compound effective in reducing joint pain.

Nettle: Rich in minerals and supports joint health; also reduces inflammation.

Ingredients:

- 2 parts dried Turmeric root
- 1 part dried Nettle leaf
- 80-proof vodka or brandy

Instructions:

1. Place the dried Turmeric root and Nettle leaf into a clean glass jar, filling it about 1/3 full with the herbs.
2. Pour vodka or brandy over the herbs until completely covered.
3. Seal the jar tightly and store in a cool, dark place for 4–6 weeks, shaking the jar daily.
4. Strain the tincture through cheesecloth and store the liquid in a dark glass bottle with a dropper.

Usage: Take 1/4 to 1/2 teaspoon 1–2 times daily to relieve joint pain and inflammation.

Source: Hewlings & Kalman, 2017

Calendula and Lavender Pain-Relief Salve

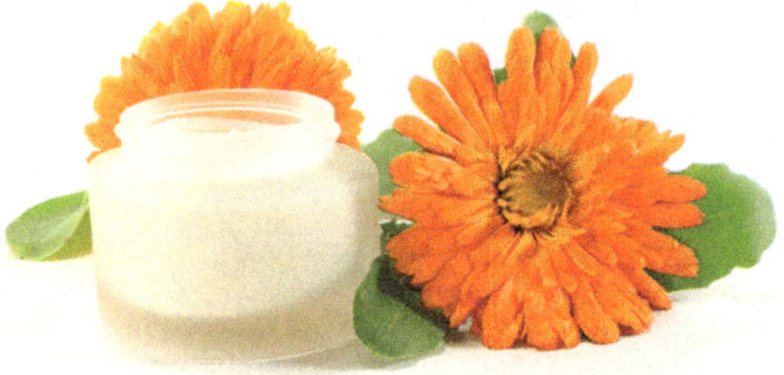

Calendula: Soothes inflammation and promotes healing.

Lavender: Provides pain relief and has calming anti-inflammatory properties.

Ingredients:

- 1/4 cup dried Calendula flowers
- 1/4 cup dried Lavender flowers
- 1 cup olive oil or coconut oil (for infusion)
- 1 oz beeswax (for thickening)
- *Optional*: 10 drops Lavender essential oil (for added pain-relief and calming effect)

Instructions:

1. In a small saucepan, combine the Calendula and Lavender with the olive or coconut oil.
2. Heat gently over low heat for about 2–3 hours to infuse the oil (without burning the herbs).
3. Strain the oil through cheesecloth or a fine mesh sieve into a clean jar.
4. In a double boiler, melt the beeswax.
5. Slowly add the strained oil to the melted beeswax, stirring well to combine.
6. Once fully blended, remove from heat and add the optional Lavender essential oil.
7. Pour the mixture into salve tins or glass jars and allow it to cool completely before capping.

Usage: Massage this salve into sore muscles and joints for pain relief. It can also be applied to minor skin irritations or areas of discomfort.

Source: Bone & Mills, 2013

Ginger and Peppermint Warming Pain Relief Salve

Ginger: Known for its anti-inflammatory and analgesic properties, Ginger helps reduce muscle and joint pain when applied topically. It also improves circulation, enhancing the warming effect.

Peppermint: Provides a cooling effect on the skin, helps relax muscles, and reduces discomfort from soreness or inflammation.

Ingredients:

- 1 cup carrier oil (such as coconut oil)
- 1 oz beeswax
- 1 tbsp Ginger powder (made by thinly slicing fresh Ginger, dehydrating until brittle, then grinding to a fine powder)
- 1 tbsp dried Peppermint leaves

Instructions:

1. Infuse the Ginger and Peppermint in the oil over low heat for 2–3 hours.
2. Strain the oil through cheesecloth.
3. Return the oil to low heat and add beeswax, stirring until melted.
4. Pour into containers and allow to cool completely.

Usage: Apply a small amount to sore muscles or joints, avoiding sensitive areas and broken skin.

Source: Ryan et al., 2011

Astragalus and Ginger Pain-Relief Tea

Astragalus: Supports immune function and reduces inflammation, helping to alleviate pain.

Ginger: A powerful anti-inflammatory that helps relieve joint and muscle pain.

Ingredients:

- 1 tsp dried Astragalus root
- 1 tsp dried Ginger root
- 1 cup hot water

Instructions:

1. Combine the Astragalus and Ginger in a tea infuser or directly into a cup.
2. Pour hot water over the herbs and steep for 10–15 minutes.
3. Strain the herbs or remove the infuser, and drink while warm.

Usage: Drink 1–2 cups daily to support pain relief and reduce inflammation.

Source: Ryan et al., 2011

Skin, Hair, and Beauty

Glowing skin and beautiful hair are not only signs of outward beauty, but also reflections of inner health and vitality. Explore this collection of herbal remedies designed to nourish and support the skin and hair from the inside out.

Calendula and Lavender Skin Soothing Salve

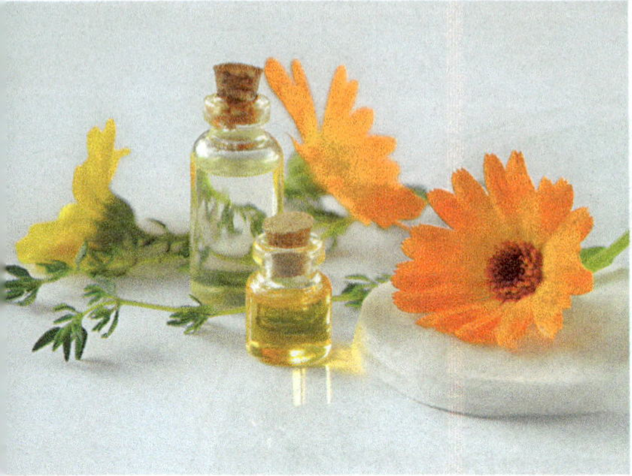

Calendula is renowned for its skin-healing properties. It has anti-inflammatory and antimicrobial effects, making it useful for minor wounds, burns, and skin irritations. Calendula can also help stimulate collagen production, supporting skin elasticity and healing.

Lavender is not only calming for the mind but also soothing for the skin. It has antimicrobial and anti-inflammatory properties and can help speed wound healing. Its gentle scent also makes it a pleasant addition to skincare preparations.

Ingredients:

- 1/4 cup dried Calendula flowers
- 1/4 cup dried Lavender flowers
- 1 cup olive oil or sweet Almond oil
- 1 oz beeswax

Instructions:

1. Infuse the herbs in the oil over low heat for 2–3 hours.
2. Strain the oil through cheesecloth.
3. Return the oil to low heat and add beeswax, stirring until melted.
4. Pour into containers and allow to cool completely.

Usage: Apply to minor skin irritations, dry skin, or minor wounds as needed.

Note: Always do a patch test before applying new products to your skin. Avoid using these products on deep or infected wounds.

Source: Bone & Mills, 2013

Rosemary and Nettle Hair Growth Salve

Rosemary has been shown to stimulate hair growth and improve circulation to the scalp. It may be as effective as minoxidil for androgenetic alopecia (male or female pattern baldness).

Nettle is rich in nutrients that support hair health, including Silica and Sulfur. It may help reduce hair loss and stimulate new growth.

Ingredients:

- 1 cup carrier oil (like Jojoba or coconut oil)
- 1 oz Beeswax
- 2 tbsp dried Rosemary leaves
- 2 tbsp dried Nettle leaves
- 10 drops Rosemary essential oil (optional)

Instructions:

1. Infuse Rosemary and Nettle in the carrier oil over low heat for 2–3 hours
2. Strain through cheesecloth
3. Return oil to low heat, add beeswax and stir until melted
4. Add essential oil if using
5. Pour into containers and let cool completely

Usage: Massage a small amount into scalp before bed or leave in for several hours before washing hair. Use 3–4 times per week.

Note: For both preparations, be aware that Rosemary may darken light hair slightly over time.

Source: Bone & Mills, 2013

Chamomile and Licorice Root Brightening Face Mask

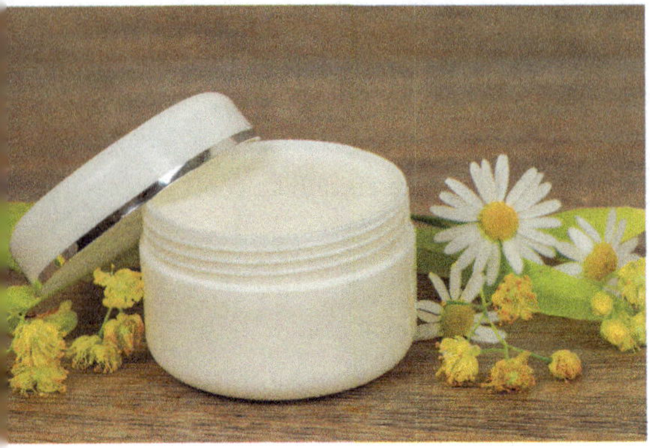

Chamomile has anti-inflammatory and antioxidant properties that can soothe and protect the skin. It may also help even out skin tone and reduce the appearance of dark spots.

Licorice root contains glabridin, a compound that may inhibit the production of melanin, potentially helping to lighten dark spots and even out skin tone.

Ingredients:

- 2 tbsp dried Chamomile flowers
- 1 tbsp Licorice root powder (made by cutting dried Licorice root into small pieces and grinding in a spice grinder or mortar and pestle until finely powdered)
- 3 tbsp raw honey
- 1 tbsp plain yogurt

Instructions:

1. Grind the Chamomile flowers into a fine powder.
2. Mix all ingredients together to form a paste.

Usage: Apply to clean skin, avoiding the eye area. Leave on for 15–20 minutes, then rinse with warm water. Use 1–2 times per week.

Note: Always do a patch test before using new skincare products. Those with hormone-sensitive conditions should avoid using Licorice root products regularly.

Source: Dai et al., 2022

Aloe Vera and Turmeric Acne-Fighting Gel

Aloe Vera is well-known for its skin-soothing properties. It has anti-inflammatory effects and can help speed wound healing, making it useful for acne-prone skin.

Turmeric has powerful anti-inflammatory and antimicrobial properties. When used topically, it may help reduce acne and even out skin tone.

Ingredients:

- 1/4 cup pure Aloe Vera gel (made by selecting a mature outer leaf, washing thoroughly, removing serrated edges, slicing lengthwise, then gently scraping the clear inner gel with a spoon)
- 1/2 tsp Turmeric powder (made by peeling fresh Turmeric root, thinly slicing, drying until brittle, then grinding to a fine powder in a spice grinder)
- 2 drops Tea Tree essential oil (optional, for additional antimicrobial effects)

Instructions:

1. Mix all ingredients thoroughly.
2. Store in a clean, airtight container in the refrigerator.

Usage: Apply a thin layer to cleansed skin as a spot treatment or all over the face, avoiding the eye area. Leave on for 15–20 minutes, then rinse. Use daily or as needed.

Note: Turmeric can stain skin and clothing. Usually, a gentle cleanser can remove the yellow tint on skin within an hour. Always conduct a patch test prior to use.

Source: Jurenka, 2009

Aloe Vera and Lavender Hair Conditioner

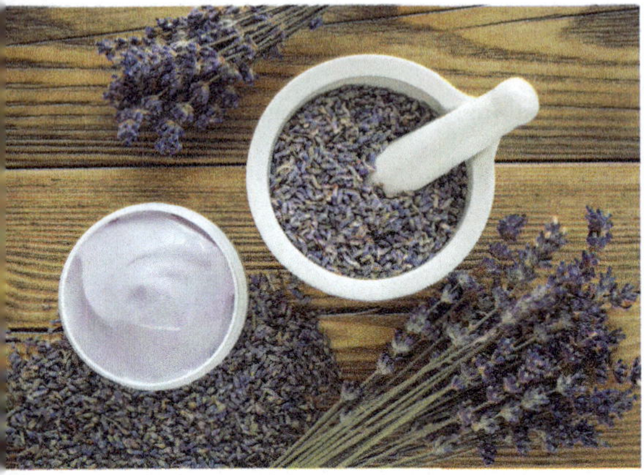

Aloe Vera: Hydrates and soothes the scalp, while promoting hair growth and reducing inflammation.

Lavender: Supports healthy hair growth and calms the scalp, reducing itchiness and dryness.

Ingredients:

- 1/4 cup Aloe Vera gel (extracted from fresh Aloe Vera leaves by cutting off the spiny edges, removing the clear inner gel, and blending until smooth)
- 5 drops Lavender tincture
- 1 tbsp coconut oil

Instructions:

1. Mix Aloe Vera gel, Lavender tincture, and coconut oil in a bowl until well combined.
2. Store the mixture in a clean, airtight container.

Usage: Apply to the scalp and hair after shampooing. Leave in for 15–20 minutes, then rinse with warm water. Use weekly for best results.

Source: Williamson, 2001

Sleep Support and Relaxation

Restful, restorative sleep is the foundation for overall well-being, yet many struggle to achieve it. This collection of herbal remedies offers a natural approach to promoting relaxation, reducing stress and anxiety, and supporting healthy sleep patterns.

Valerian and Passionflower Sleep Well Tincture

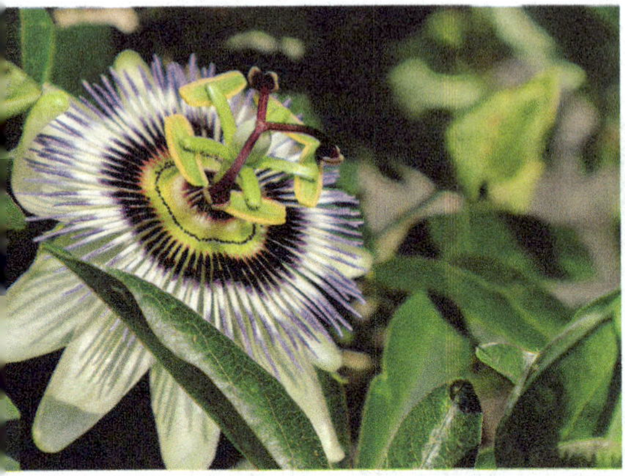

Valerian has been used for centuries as a sleep aid. It may help reduce the time it takes to fall asleep and improve sleep quality. Valerian works by increasing levels of gamma-aminobutyric acid (GABA), a neurotransmitter that promotes relaxation.

Passionflower has mild sedative effects and may help reduce anxiety. People often combine it with other herbs that promote sleep for a synergistic effect.

Ingredients:

- 2 parts dried Valerian root
- 1 part dried Passionflower aerial parts (leaves, stems, and flowers)
- 80-proof vodka or brandy

Instructions:

1. Fill a clean glass jar 1/3 full with the herbs.
2. Pour alcohol over the herbs until completely covered.
3. Seal the jar and store in a cool, dark place for 4–6 weeks, shaking daily.
4. Strain through cheesecloth and store in a dark glass bottle.

Usage: Take 1/4 to 1/2 teaspoon 30 minutes before bedtime to support sleep.

Note: Valerian can cause drowsiness and should not be combined with sedative medications or alcohol. Some people may experience a stimulant effect from Valerian. If this occurs, discontinue use.

Source: Akhondzadeh et al., 2002

Chamomile and Lemon Balm Relaxation Tea

Chamomile is well-known for its calming properties. It contains apigenin, a compound that binds to certain receptors in the brain, potentially promoting sleepiness and reducing insomnia.

Lemon Balm has mild sedative effects and can help reduce anxiety and promote relaxation. People often use it to enhance the quality of their sleep and lessen disturbances caused by stress.

Ingredients:

- 1 tsp dried Chamomile flowers
- 1 tsp dried Lemon Balm
- 1 cup hot water
- Honey to taste (optional)

Instructions:

1. Combine herbs in a tea infuser or bag.
2. Pour hot water over the herbs and steep for 5–10 minutes.
3. Remove herbs, add honey if desired, and drink.

Usage: Drink 1 cup 30–60 minutes before bedtime to promote relaxation and support sleep.

Note: Those with ragweed allergies may be sensitive to Chamomile. Lemon Balm may interact with thyroid medications and sedatives.

Source: Cohen et al., 1964

Lavender and Hops Sleep Support Tea

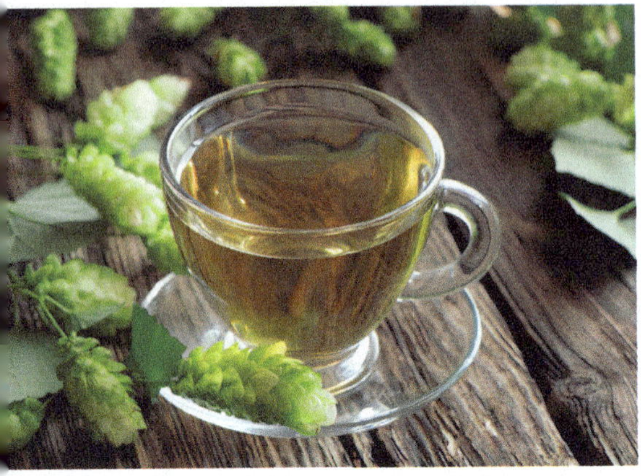

Lavender: Promotes relaxation and reduces anxiety, helping you unwind before sleep.

Hops: Known for its mild sedative properties, it helps induce sleep and reduce restlessness.

Ingredients:

- 1 tsp dried Lavender flowers
- 1 tsp dried Hops flowers
- 1 cup hot water
- Honey to taste (optional)

Instructions:

1. Place the Lavender and Hops in a tea infuser or directly into a cup.
2. Pour hot water over the herbs and allow them to steep for 5–10 minutes.
3. Remove the infuser or strain the herbs from the cup.
4. Add honey for sweetness, if desired.

Usage: Drink 1 cup 30–60 minutes before bedtime to help relax and improve sleep quality.

Source: Franco et al., 2012

Lavender and Lemon Balm Relaxation Tea

Lavender: Calms the nervous system and helps reduce anxiety, promoting better sleep.

Lemon Balm: Reduces stress and enhances relaxation, improving sleep quality.

Ingredients:

- 1 tsp dried Lavender flowers
- 1 tsp dried Lemon Balm leaves
- 1 cup hot water

Instructions:

1. Place the Lavender flowers, and Lemon Balm leaves into a tea infuser or directly into a cup.
2. Pour hot water over the herbs and steep for 5–10 minutes.
3. Remove the infuser or strain the herbs, and drink while warm.

Usage: Drink 1 cup 30 minutes before bedtime to help promote restful sleep.

Source: Williamson, 2001

Valerian and Lemon Balm Sleep Tincture

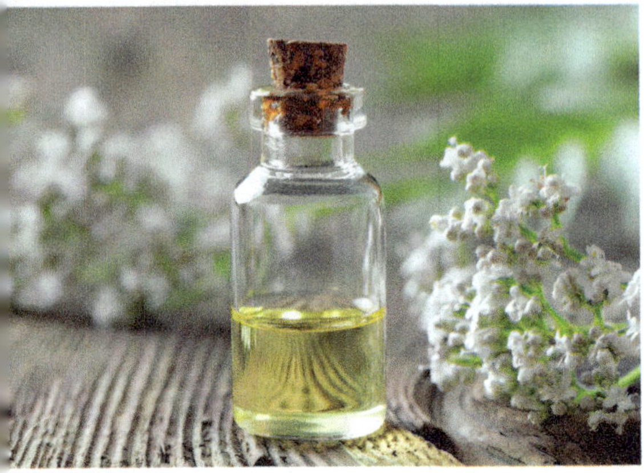

Valerian: Acts as a natural sedative, helping reduce the time it takes to fall asleep and improving sleep quality.

Lemon Balm: Calms the mind and helps reduce anxiety, promoting relaxation before bed.

Ingredients:

- 2 parts dried Valerian root
- 1 part dried Lemon Balm leaves
- 80-proof vodka or brandy

Instructions:

1. Fill a clean glass jar 1/3 full with the herbs.
2. Pour alcohol over the herbs until fully submerged.
3. Seal the jar and store it in a cool, dark place for 4–6 weeks, shaking daily.
4. Strain the mixture through cheesecloth and store it in a dark glass bottle.

Usage: Take 1/4 to 1/2 teaspoon 30 minutes before bedtime to support deep, restful sleep.

Source: Cohen et al., 1964

Stress and Anxiety Reduction

In our fast-paced, high-stress world, finding effective ways to manage anxiety and reduce stress is essential for maintaining overall health and well-being. This collection of herbal remedies offers a natural approach to calming the mind and promoting a sense of inner peace.

Lemon Balm and Passionflower Stress and Sleep Support Tea

Lemon Balm is known for its calming effects on the nervous system and has been shown to reduce stress and anxiety while promoting restful sleep.

Passionflower helps ease anxiety and insomnia through its gentle sedative properties, helping to quiet an overactive mind.

Ingredients:

- 1 tsp dried Lemon Balm leaves
- 1 tsp dried Passionflower aerial parts
- Optional: 1/2 tsp dried Chamomile flowers for enhanced relaxation
- 1 cup hot water
- Honey to taste (optional)

Instructions:

1. Place Lemon Balm and Passionflower (and Chamomile if using) in a tea infuser or bag
2. Pour hot water over herbs
3. Cover and steep for 10 minutes
4. Remove herbs and add honey if desired

Usage: Drink 1 cup 30–60 minutes before bedtime to promote relaxation and restful sleep.

Note: Both herbs are generally safe, but may cause drowsiness. Do not drive or operate machinery after consuming. If taking prescription sedatives or antianxiety medications, consult your healthcare provider before use.

Source: Cohen et al., 1964

St. John's Wort and Lemon Balm Mood Support Tea

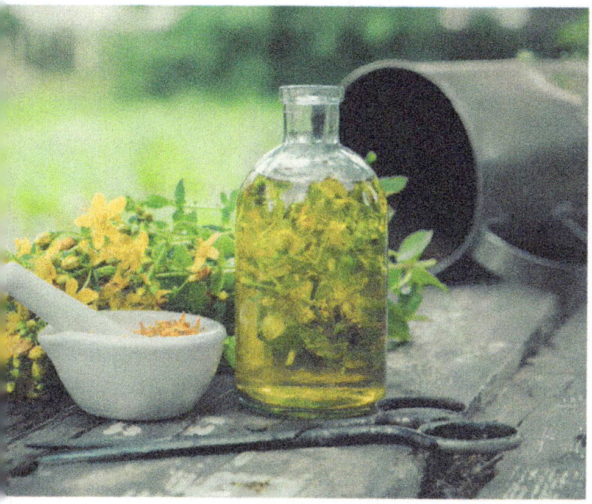

St. John's Wort contains compounds like hypericin that help regulate neurotransmitters involved in mood regulation. Studies have shown it may help with mild to moderate depression and anxiety.

Lemon Balm has been shown to have calming effects and may help reduce symptoms of anxiety and stress. It works by modulating GABA, a neurotransmitter that promotes relaxation.

Ingredients:

- 1 tsp dried St. John's Wort aerial parts
- 1 tsp dried Lemon Balm leaves
- 1 cup hot water
- Honey to taste (optional)

Instructions:

1. Combine herbs in a tea infuser or bag
2. Pour hot water over the herbs and steep for 10 minutes
3. Strain and drink

Usage: Drink 1–2 cups daily to support emotional wellbeing and stress relief.

Note: St. John's Wort can interact with many medications including antidepressants, birth control pills, and blood thinners. It may also cause photosensitivity. Consult a healthcare provider before use, especially if taking any medications. Lemon balm may interact with thyroid medications and sedatives.

Source: Cohen et al., 1964

Lavender and Passionflower Calming Tincture

Lavender: Calms the nervous system and helps reduce stress and anxiety.

Passionflower: Has mild sedative properties and is often used to reduce anxiety and promote restful sleep.

Ingredients:

- 2 parts dried Lavender flowers
- 1 part dried Passionflower aerial parts
- 80-proof vodka or brandy

Instructions:

1. Place the dried Lavender and Passionflower into a clean glass jar, filling it about 1/3 full with the herbs.
2. Pour the vodka or brandy over the herbs, ensuring they are completely submerged.
3. Seal the jar tightly and store in a cool, dark place for 4–6 weeks, shaking the jar daily.
4. After 4–6 weeks, strain the tincture through cheesecloth or a fine mesh sieve and transfer the liquid into a dark glass bottle with a dropper.

Usage: Take 1/4 to 1/2 teaspoon 1–2 times daily for calming effects, especially before bedtime or during periods of anxiety.

Source: Akhondzadeh et al., 2002

Rhodiola and Holy Basil Stress-Relief Tincture

Rhodiola: Known for its adaptogenic properties, Rhodiola helps the body adapt to stress and reduces mental and physical fatigue.

Holy Basil: Another adaptogen, it helps balance stress hormones and calms the nervous system, making it excellent for relieving anxiety.

Ingredients:

- 2 parts dried Rhodiola root
- 1 part dried Holy Basil leaves
- 80-proof vodka or brandy

Instructions:

1. Place the dried Rhodiola and Holy Basil into a clean glass jar, filling it about 1/3 full with the herbs.
2. Pour the vodka or brandy over the herbs, ensuring they are fully submerged.
3. Seal the jar tightly and store in a cool, dark place for 4–6 weeks, shaking daily.
4. After 4–6 weeks, strain the tincture through cheesecloth and transfer the liquid to a dark glass bottle with a dropper.

Usage: Take 1/4 to 1/2 teaspoon 1–2 times daily to help manage stress and anxiety.

Source: Ishaque et al., 2012

Ashwagandha and Lemon Balm Anti-Stress Tincture

Ashwagandha: Helps the body adapt to stress and reduces cortisol levels, promoting calmness.

Lemon Balm: Relieves anxiety and helps relax the mind, reducing feelings of stress.

Ingredients:

- 2 parts dried Ashwagandha root
- 1 part dried Lemon Balm leaves
- 80-proof vodka or brandy

Instructions:

1. Fill a clean glass jar 1/3 full with the herbs.
2. Pour alcohol over the herbs until fully covered.
3. Seal the jar and store in a cool, dark place for 4–6 weeks, shaking daily.
4. Strain the mixture through cheesecloth and store it in a dark glass bottle with a dropper.

Usage: Take 1/4 to 1/2 teaspoon 1–2 times daily to relieve stress and anxiety.

Source: Williamson, 2001

Women's Health

Supporting women's health involves addressing the unique challenges that arise throughout different life stages. Herbal remedies in this therapeutic category focus on balancing hormones, easing menstrual and menopausal symptoms, and promoting overall reproductive health.

Ashwagandha and Fennel Women's Balance Tea

Ashwagandha: Helps balance stress hormones and promotes overall well-being, making it great for reducing stress that can impact hormonal health.

Fennel: Aids in relieving menstrual cramps and supports hormonal balance, while also promoting digestive health.

Ingredients:

- 1 tsp dried Ashwagandha root
- 1 tsp dried Fennel seeds
- 1 cup hot water

Instructions:

1. Place the dried Ashwagandha and Fennel into a tea infuser or directly into a cup.
2. Pour hot water over the herbs and steep for 10–15 minutes.
3. Strain the herbs or remove the infuser, and drink while warm.

Usage: Drink 1–2 cups daily to support hormonal balance, reduce stress, and relieve menstrual discomfort.

Source: Williamson, 2001

Ashwagandha and St. John's Wort Hormone Balance Tincture

Ashwagandha is an adaptogenic herb that may help balance hormones and reduce stress, which can impact women's health.

St. John's Wort is known for its mood-balancing properties and may help alleviate symptoms of PMS and menopause.

Ingredients:

- 2 parts dried Ashwagandha root
- 1 part dried St. John's Wort flowering tops
- 80-proof vodka or brandy

Instructions:

1. Fill a clean glass jar 1/3 full with the herbs.
2. Pour alcohol over the herbs until completely covered.
3. Seal the jar and store in a cool, dark place for 4–6 weeks, shaking daily.
4. Strain through cheesecloth and store in a dark glass bottle.

Usage: Take 1/4 to 1/2 teaspoon 1–2 times daily to support hormone balance.

Note: St. John's Wort may interact with many medications, including birth control. Consult a healthcare provider before use, especially if you're taking any medications.

Source: Linde et al., 2008

Licorice and Fennel Menstrual Support Tea

Licorice may help balance hormones and reduce inflammation associated with menstrual discomfort.

Fennel can help alleviate menstrual cramps and support digestive health during menstruation.

Ingredients:

- 1 tsp dried Licorice root
- 1 tsp Fennel seeds
- 1 cup hot water

Instructions:

1. Combine herbs in a tea infuser or bag.
2. Pour hot water over the herbs and steep for 10 minutes.
3. Strain and drink.

Usage: Drink 1 cup daily during the week before and during menstruation.

Note: Licorice should not be used by those with high blood pressure, kidney disease, or during pregnancy. Do not use for more than 4–6 weeks without consulting a healthcare provider.

Source: Williamson, 2001

Lavender and Chamomile Menopause Tea

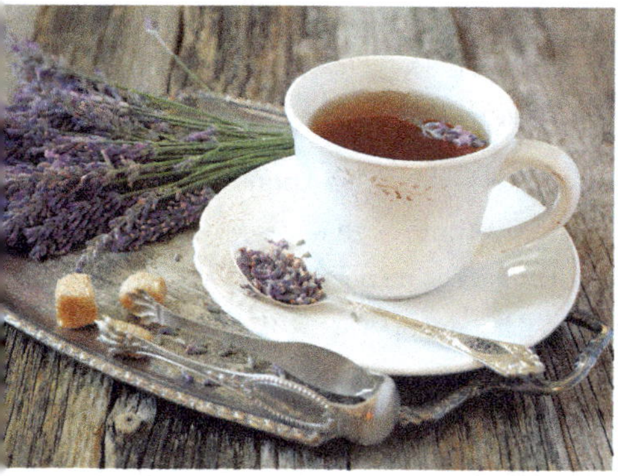

Lavender can help reduce stress and promote relaxation, which may alleviate some symptoms of menopause.

Chamomile may help reduce hot flashes and improve sleep quality during menopause.

Ingredients:

- 1 part dried Lavender flowers
- 1 part dried Chamomile flowers
- Honey (optional)

Instructions:

1. Mix the dried herbs together.
2. Use 1 tsp of the blend per cup of hot water.
3. Steep for 5–10 minutes, strain, and add honey if desired.

Usage: Drink 1–2 cups daily to support relaxation and alleviate menopausal symptoms.

Note: Those with ragweed allergies may be sensitive to Chamomile.

Source: Dai et al., 2022

Fennel and Lemon Balm Women's Health Tincture

Fennel: Supports hormonal balance, helps relieve menstrual cramps, and improves reproductive health.

Lemon Balm: Calms the nervous system, reduces stress, and helps regulate hormones, especially during menstruation or menopause.

Ingredients:

- 2 parts dried Fennel seeds
- 1 part dried Lemon Balm leaves
- 80-proof vodka or brandy

Instructions:

1. Place the dried Fennel seeds and Lemon Balm leaves into a clean glass jar, filling it about 1/3 full with the herbs.
2. Pour vodka or brandy over the herbs, ensuring they are fully submerged.
3. Seal the jar tightly and store in a cool, dark place for 4–6 weeks, shaking daily.
4. After 4–6 weeks, strain the tincture through cheesecloth and transfer it into a dark glass bottle with a dropper.

Usage: Take 1/4 to 1/2 teaspoon 1–2 times daily to support hormonal balance and reduce menstrual discomfort.

Source: Cohen et al., 1964

Exploring Nature's Pharmacy for Well-Being

Herbal remedies offer a natural way to support health throughout all stages of life. Use them responsibly, starting with the lowest dose and observing the body's response, despite their power. Herbal medicine is not universally applicable, so it's crucial to pay attention to your body's needs and seek advice from a healthcare practitioner when necessary. As you continue to learn and experiment with herbs, you'll find a vast and fascinating world that can empower your path to vibrant health.

CHAPTER 7:
EMERGING TRENDS IN HERBAL MEDICINE

Herbal medicine has a rich history dating back thousands of years, but it is far from a static field. As scientific understanding advances and global influences shape our health practices, herbal medicine is undergoing a transformation. This chapter delves into the latest innovations and emerging trends in herbal medicine, emphasizing their potential integration into home-based herbal practices. From personalized formulations to sustainable sourcing, from adaptogens to innovative delivery methods, these trends represent the future of herbal medicine. For anyone interested in making herbal remedies at home, staying informed about these trends is essential for creating effective, sustainable, and cutting-edge preparations.

Personalized Herbal Medicine

One of the most exciting trends in herbal medicine is the move towards personalized formulations. Advances in genomics and data analysis are making it possible to tailor herbal remedies to an individual's unique constitution, health history, and wellness goals. Businesses such as Care/of and Vitagene are currently utilizing questionnaires and DNA tests to develop personalized supplement regimens, and herbal medicine could adopt similar strategies (Thomford et al., 2018).

For example, an individual with a genetic predisposition to inflammation might benefit from a personalized blend of anti-inflammatory herbs like Turmeric and Ginger. We could recommend a custom formula featuring adaptogens like Ashwagandha and Holy Basil, combined with nervines like Passionflower and Lemon Balm, for someone struggling with stress and anxiety. As research in this area progresses, home herbalists may be able to access tools and resources to help them create personalized remedies tailored to their specific needs.

Scientific Validation and Integration

Another major trend in herbal medicine is the increasing scientific validation of traditional herbal knowledge. Rigorous studies are confirming the efficacy of many herbs for a variety of health conditions, from Echinacea for immune support (Weber et al., 2005) to St. John's Wort for mild to moderate depression (Laakmann et al., 1998). This research not only validates traditional uses but also helps to identify optimal dosages, preparation methods, and potential interactions or contraindications.

As this body of research grows, it is influencing the integration of herbal medicine into mainstream healthcare. Many hospitals and clinics now offer integrative medicine programs that incorporate herbal remedies alongside conventional treatments (Onyambu, 2019). For home herbalists, this trend underscores the importance of staying informed about the latest scientific findings. Basing herbal preparations on scientifically validated information can help ensure safety and effectiveness.

Sustainability and Ethical Sourcing

As the demand for herbal products grows, sustainability and ethical sourcing are becoming increasingly important considerations. Many popular herbs, such as Goldenseal and Echinacea, have been overharvested from the wild, leading to dwindling populations (Weber et al., 2005). Other herbs, like Rhodiola, are primarily wild-harvested from fragile ecosystems that are vulnerable to disruption (Li et al., 2017). Cultivating herbs domestically or sourcing from certified sustainable wildcrafters can help alleviate these pressures.

Home herbalists can contribute to sustainability efforts by growing their own herbs using organic methods. Herbs like Peppermint, Calendula, and Chamomile are easy to grow in a home garden, providing a fresh, sustainable supply for herbal preparations. When purchasing herbs, look for organic, fair trade, or sustainably wild-crafted certifications. Supporting ethical and sustainable herb production helps ensure the long-term viability of herbal medicine.

Globalization of Traditional Remedies

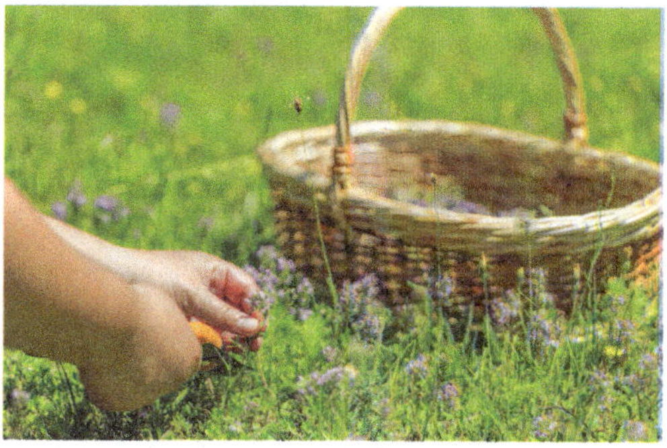

The globalization of herbal medicine is making a wider variety of traditional remedies available to home herbalists. Many health food stores and online retailers now carry herbs from various cultural traditions, such as Ashwagandha from Ayurveda or Astragalus (Foster & Johnson 2006). Globalization is also shaping the use of these herbs, incorporating many into modern formulations and delivery methods. However, increased global demand has put many traditional medicinal herbs at risk of overharvesting and habitat loss.

For home herbalists, this trend opens up exciting possibilities for exploring new herbs and traditional healing practices. However, it's important to approach these herbs with respect and understanding of their cultural context. Learning about the traditional preparation methods and uses of these herbs can help guide their incorporation into modern herbal practice. It's also crucial to source these herbs from reputable suppliers who respect traditional knowledge and engage in fair trade practices.

Adaptogens and Stress Relief

In our fast-paced, high-stress modern world, adaptogens are emerging as a popular solution for stress management and resilience. Adaptogens are a class of herbs that help the body adapt to stress, supporting overall well-being and vitality (Panossian & Wikman, 2010). Some of the most popular adaptogens include Ashwagandha, Rhodiola, Holy Basil, and Astragalus.

You can easily incorporate Adaptogens into home herbal remedies for stress relief. You can steep Ashwagandha, Holy Basil, and Licorice root in hot water to create a simple Adaptogenic tea blend that you can enjoy daily. You can also prepare Adaptogenic herbs as tinctures, capsules, or incorporate them into smoothies and other foods. By supporting the body's resilience to stress, these herbs can be valuable allies in maintaining overall health and well-being.

Innovation in Delivery Methods

Innovation in delivery methods is making herbal remedies more convenient, effective, and accessible. One emerging trend is the use of herbal extracts in novel formats like gummies, lozenges, and effervescent powders. These formats can make herbs like Elderberry or Echinacea more palatable and easier to take regularly for immune support.

Another area of innovation is in topical applications. Herbs like Calendula and Turmeric are being incorporated into creams, balms, and patches for localized pain relief and skin health. Transdermal patches, in particular, are an emerging method for delivering herbal compounds steadily over time, which may improve bioavailability and efficacy (Cheng et al., 2020).

Home herbalists can experiment with these innovative delivery methods to create their own modern herbal remedies. For example, you could create an immune-supportive Elderberry gummy by blending Elderberry syrup with gelatin and honey. Or, you could infuse oil with Calendula and Lavender to create a soothing balm for skin irritations. By staying informed about these innovations, home herbalists can expand their herbal toolkit and create remedies that are effective, convenient, and enjoyable to use.

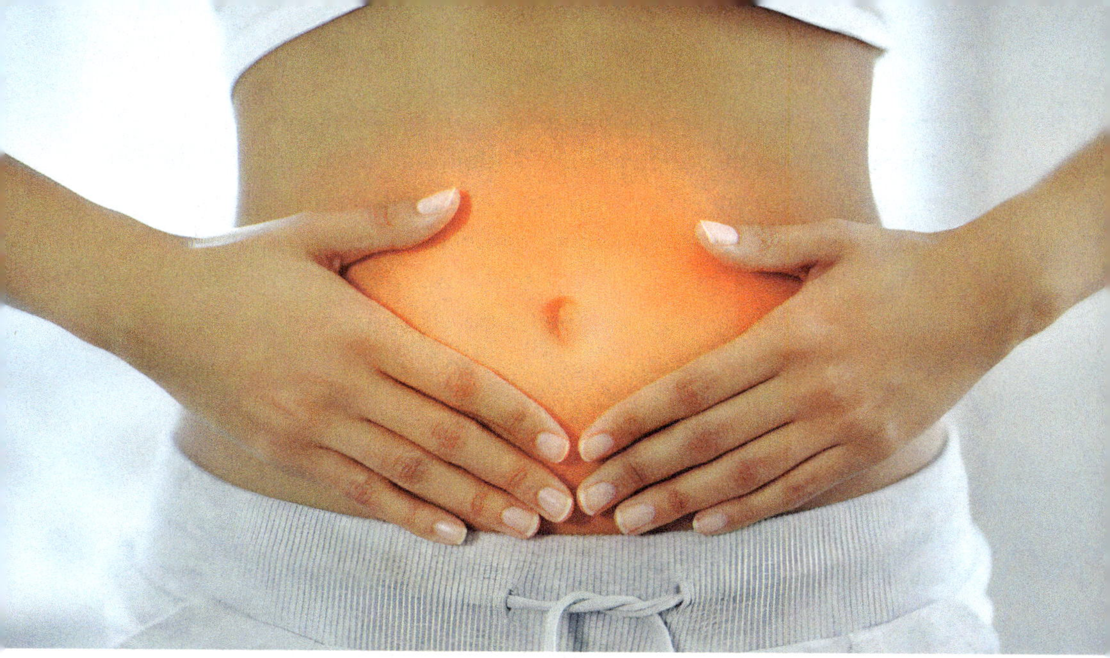

Focus on Gut Health

Gut health is emerging as a key focus in herbal medicine, reflecting the growing understanding of the gut's central role in overall health and well-being. Researchers have linked imbalances in the gut microbiome to a wide range of health issues, including digestive disorders, autoimmune diseases, allergies, and even mental health concerns (Lynch & Pedersen, 2016).

Modern research is validating the effectiveness of many herbs used traditionally to support gut health. For instance, studies have demonstrated the potential of Licorice root to prevent and heal gastric ulcers (Wahab et al., 2021). Chamomile and Peppermint are well-known for their ability to soothe digestive discomfort and calm intestinal spasms (Foster & Johnson, 2006). Researchers have found that Burdock root and Dandelion root, traditionally used as digestive bitters, stimulate digestive secretions and support liver function (Petkova et al., 2021).

Home herbalists can incorporate these gut-supportive herbs into their wellness routines in various ways. A daily tea blend of Peppermint, Chamomile, and Fennel can help soothe digestion and reduce bloating. A Burdock and Dandelion tincture taken before meals can stimulate digestive secretions and improve nutrient absorption. By supporting gut health with herbal remedies, home herbalists can promote overall well-being and resilience.

Herbal Remedies for Chronic Conditions

As chronic diseases become increasingly prevalent, more people are turning to herbal medicine for long-term management and support. People often use herbs as a complement to conventional treatments to manage conditions such as diabetes, cardiovascular disease, autoimmune disorders, and more.

For example, Turmeric has been traditionally used in Ayurvedic medicine to treat inflammation and joint pain, and modern research has confirmed its anti-inflammatory and pain-reducing properties, particularly in conditions like osteoarthritis (Jurenka, 2009). Clinical trials have demonstrated the effectiveness of St. John's Wort, a traditional European remedy for mood disorders, for mild to moderate depression (Laakmann et al., 1998). Holy Basil, another Ayurvedic herb, has been traditionally used for stress and anxiety, and recent studies validate its adaptogenic properties in helping the body manage stress responses (Cohen, 2014).

For home herbalists, creating long-term herbal treatment plans for chronic conditions requires careful research and, ideally, guidance from a qualified healthcare practitioner. It's important to understand potential herb-drug interactions and to monitor health markers regularly. However, with proper precautions, herbal remedies can be a valuable tool in managing chronic diseases and supporting overall health.

CBD and Cannabis-Based Products

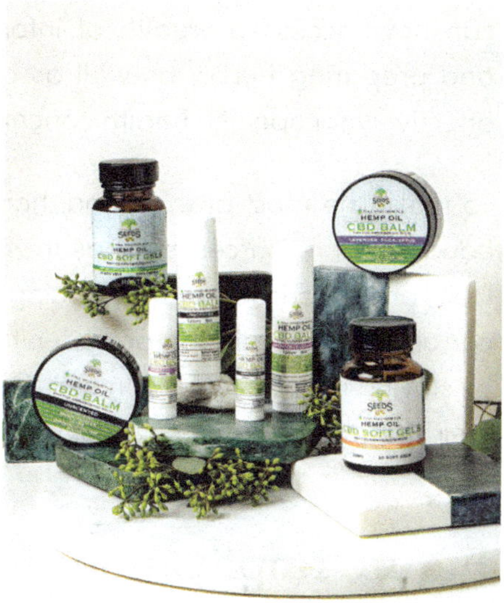

The legalization of cannabis in many areas has led to a surge of interest in CBD (cannabidiol) and other cannabis-based products for health and wellness. Cannabis contains CBD, a non-psychoactive compound that has demonstrated potential benefits for pain, anxiety, sleep, and other conditions (Blessing et al., 2015).

As cannabis laws continue to evolve, CBD products are becoming more widely available, from oils and tinctures to edibles and topicals. Some herbalists are also exploring the potential of other cannabis compounds, like CBG (cannabigerol) and CBN (cannabinol) as well as full-spectrum cannabis preparations.

For home herbalists interested in working with cannabis-based products, it's crucial to stay informed about the legal status of cannabis in your area. It's also important to source CBD and other cannabis products from reputable suppliers who provide third-party lab testing results to ensure quality and potency. When incorporating cannabis-based products into herbal remedies, start with low doses and monitor the effects carefully.

Herbal Education and Consumer Empowerment

One of the most exciting trends in herbal medicine is the growing availability of herbal education resources and the resulting empowerment of consumers. Online courses, workshops, blogs, and social media are making it easier than ever for people to learn about herbs and make informed decisions about their health.

This trend is democratizing herbal knowledge and enabling more people to take an active role in their health and well-being. Home herbalists can now access a wealth of information about growing, harvesting, and preparing herbs, as well as guidance on using herbs safely and effectively for specific health concerns.

To make the most of this trend, home herbalists can seek out reputable educational resources, such as those offered by the American Herbalists Guild or the Herbal Academy. Joining local herb clubs or online communities can also provide valuable opportunities for learning and sharing knowledge. By staying informed and connected, home herbalists can continue to grow their skills and confidence in using herbs for health and wellness.

Future Implications

As these trends continue to shape the field of herbal medicine, they hold exciting implications for the future of home herbalism. Personalized and scientifically validated herbal remedies may become increasingly accessible, enabling home herbalists to create targeted, effective formulations for their unique needs. Sustainable and ethical sourcing practices may become the norm, ensuring a reliable supply of high-quality herbs for generations to come.

At the same time, these trends may also present challenges for home herbalists. As herbal medicine becomes more mainstream and regulated, it may become harder for home herbalists to access certain herbs or make certain preparations. Staying informed about changes in regulations and industry standards will be crucial for navigating this evolving landscape.

The collective actions and choices of herbalists, consumers, and policymakers will ultimately shape the future of herbal medicine. By staying informed, engaged, and proactive, home herbalists can help steer this future in a direction that prioritizes safety, efficacy, sustainability, and accessibility. The trends outlined in this chapter provide a roadmap for this journey, offering exciting opportunities for growth, innovation, and empowerment in the world of home herbalism.

CONCLUSION

As we conclude our exploration of herbal medicine, I hope you feel empowered to continue your journey with herbs. You've learned about 25 of the most versatile herbs—how to select quality herbs, create effective preparations, and use them safely for wellness and healing.

Remember, this is just the beginning. To support your ongoing learning, we've included additional **resources** at the end of this book:

Glossary: A comprehensive guide to herbal medicine terminology, defining over 20 essential concepts and technical terms used throughout the field.

Resources: A carefully curated collection of trusted suppliers, educational programs, identification tools, and community platforms, including:

The following resources provide a solid foundation for continuing your herbal medicine journey, whether you're growing, wildcrafting, or purchasing herbs for your practice:

- 9 verified herbal suppliers
- 11 quality herbal product manufacturers
- 3 reliable plant identification apps
- 10 educational institutions and programs
- 4 professional journals
- Multiple community platforms and support resources

Plant Monographs: Detailed profiles of all 25 featured herbs, each including:

- Botanical information
- Native habitat and growing conditions
- Therapeutic properties
- Traditional and modern uses
- Safety considerations
- Dosage guidelines
- Contraindications and interactions

As you incorporate herbs into your life, listen to your body, start slowly, and be patient. While herbs are powerful allies, they aren't a substitute for professional medical care. Always consult with a healthcare provider, especially if you have serious health conditions or are taking medications.

The path of herbal medicine is one of empowerment, connection, and lifelong learning. By working with plants, we support our health and cultivate a deeper relationship with the natural world, becoming part of a rich tradition that recognizes the Earth's healing power.

Keep exploring, learning, and connecting with plants. May they help you achieve optimal health and well-being, and inspire you to protect and promote their wisdom.

APPENDIX I: PLANT MONOGRAPHS

Aloe Vera

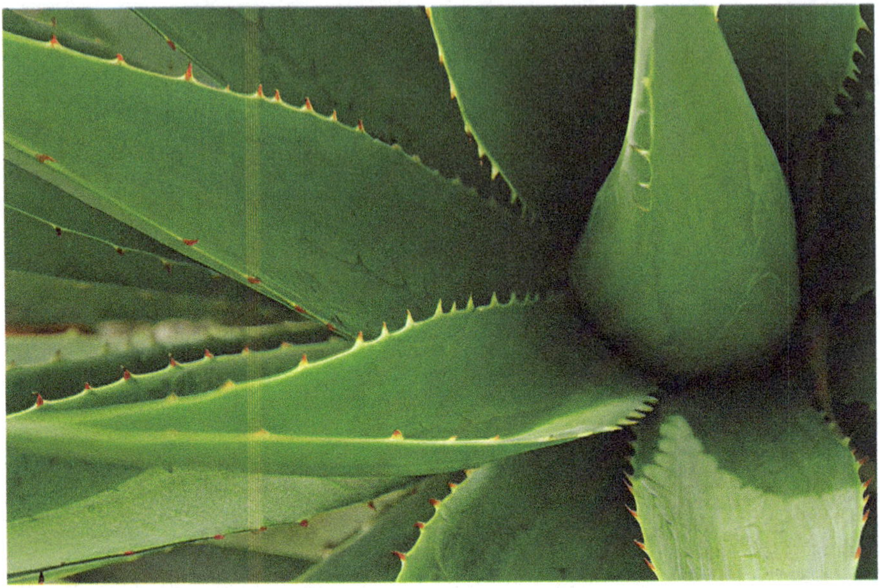

Botanical Information

Scientific Name: *Aloe barbadensis miller*

Plant Description: Aloe Vera is a succulent perennial characterized by its thick, fleshy, lance-shaped leaves that grow in a rosette pattern. The leaves are gray-green in color and have serrated edges with small white teeth. Mature plants can reach 60–100 cm in height and produce tall spikes bearing yellow or orange tubular flowers.

Native Region: Believed to have originated in the Arabian Peninsula, Aloe Vera is now widely cultivated in tropical and subtropical regions worldwide.

Habitat: Aloe Vera thrives in arid and semi-arid environments, often found growing in rocky or sandy soils with good drainage. It adapts to endure drought conditions and necessitates minimal rainfall.

Plant Parts Used: The clear, gel-like substance found in the inner part of the leaves is the primary part used for medicinal purposes. The outer leaf rind contains a yellow sap called aloe latex, which is also used therapeutically but less frequently due to its strong laxative effects.

Therapeutic Properties

Therapeutic Actions:

- *Emollient:* Softens and soothes the skin
- *Anti-inflammatory:* Reduces inflammation both internally and topically
- *Wound healing:* Promotes the repair of damaged skin tissues
- *Demulcent:* Soothes and protects irritated or inflamed internal tissues
- *Laxative (latex):* Stimulates bowel movements

Indications:

- Burns, cuts, scrapes, and other skin injuries
- Inflammatory skin conditions such as eczema or psoriasis
- Digestive issues like heartburn, acid reflux, or ulcers
- Constipation (latex)
- Immune system support

Energetics: Aloe Vera has a cooling and moistening effect on the body. It is used to clear heat and inflammation, especially in the digestive tract and on the skin.

Safety and Dosage

Dosage:

- *Topical:* Apply pure Aloe Vera gel liberally to the affected area as needed.
- *Internal (gel):* Consume 1–2 tablespoons of Aloe Vera gel daily.
- *Internal (latex):* Take 50–200 mg of dried latex daily as a laxative. Use cautiously and do not exceed recommended doses.

Contraindications: Aloe latex should be avoided during pregnancy and breastfeeding, as it may stimulate uterine contractions and cause digestive upset in infants. Individuals with severe abdominal pain, appendicitis, or intestinal blockages should not consume aloe latex.

Interactions: Aloe Vera may enhance the blood sugar-lowering effects of diabetes medications. It may also increase the potassium-depleting effects of diuretics and laxatives.

Ashwagandha

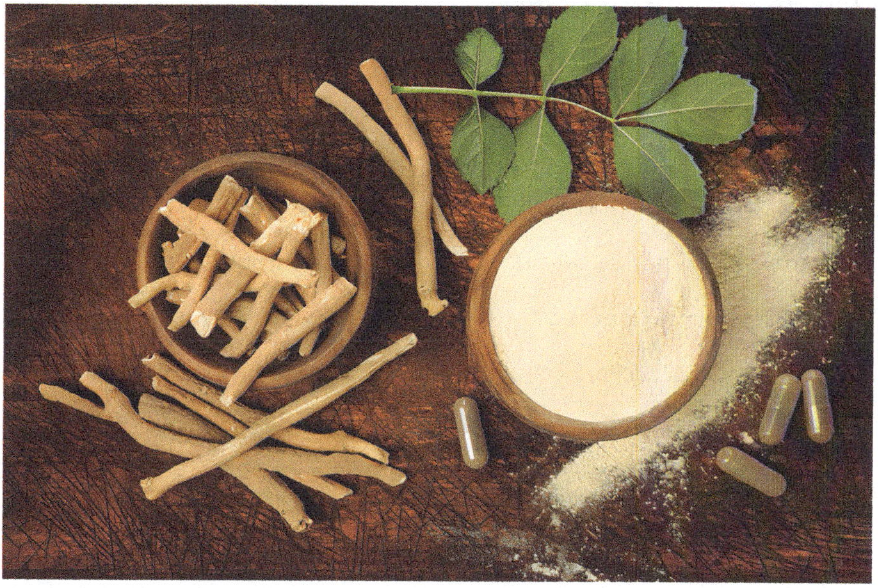

Botanical Information

Scientific Name: *Withania somnifera*

Plant Description: Ashwagandha is a small, woody shrub that typically grows to a height of 1–2 meters. It has oval-shaped leaves and bears small, greenish, or yellow flowers that develop into bright red berries. The roots are thick, fleshy, and brown in color and are the primary part used medicinally.

Native Region: Ashwagandha is native to the dry regions of India, the Middle East, and parts of North Africa.

Habitat: This hardy plant thrives in arid and semi-arid climates and is often found growing in sandy or rocky soils with good drainage. It can tolerate drought conditions and high temperatures.

Plant Parts Used: The roots are the main part used therapeutically, although the leaves and berries also contain medicinal compounds.

Therapeutic Properties

Therapeutic Actions:

- *Adaptogen:* Helps the body adapt to stress and promotes homeostasis
- *Nervine:* Calms and supports the nervous system
- *Anti-inflammatory:* Reduces inflammation throughout the body
- *Antioxidant:* Protects cells from damage caused by free radicals
- *Immunomodulator:* Regulates and supports immune function

Indications:

- Stress, anxiety, and fatigue
- Insomnia and sleep disturbances
- Cognitive decline and memory issues
- Chronic inflammation and pain
- Hormonal imbalances, particularly in women

Energetics: Ashwagandha has warming and slightly drying energy. In Ayurvedic medicine, it is considered a Rasayana herb, meaning it promotes vitality and longevity.

Safety and Dosage

Dosage:

- Powder: 1–6 grams daily, usually taken in divided doses with warm milk or water

- Tincture: 2–4 mL, taken 2–3 times daily
- Capsules: 500–1000 mg, taken 1–2 times daily

Contraindications: People with hyperthyroidism should avoid Ashwagandha as it may increase thyroid hormone levels. People with autoimmune conditions should also use it cautiously, as it may stimulate the immune system.

Interactions: Ashwagandha may enhance the effects of sedative medications, including barbiturates and benzodiazepines. It may also interact with thyroid medications and immunosuppressants.

Astragalus

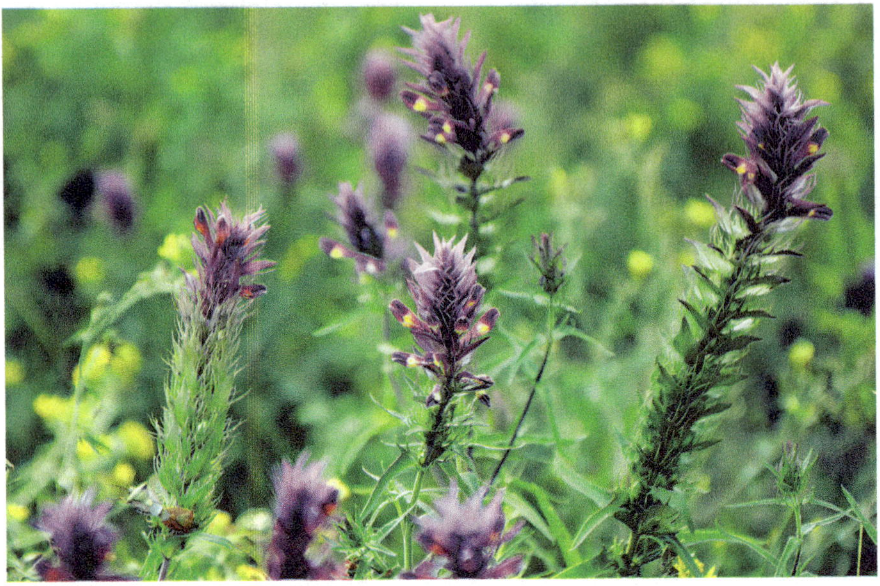

Botanical Information

Scientific Name: *Astragalus membranaceus*

Plant Description: Astragalus is a perennial herb that can grow up to 1 meter tall. It has hairy stems and pinnate leaves composed of 12–18 pairs of leaflets. The flowers are small, yellow, and arranged in clusters. The root system consists of a taproot and numerous lateral roots that are long, fibrous, and yellowish-brown in color.

Native Region: Astragalus is native to the temperate regions of the Northern Hemisphere, including China, Mongolia, and Siberia.

Habitat: This plant is commonly found growing in grassy meadows, on mountainsides, and in open woodlands. It prefers well-drained, sandy, or loamy soils and can tolerate a wide range of temperatures.

Plant Parts Used: The root is the primary part used medicinally, usually harvested from 4-year-old plants in the autumn.

Therapeutic Properties

Therapeutic Actions:

- *Adaptogen*: Helps the body adapt to stress and promotes overall well-being
- *Immunomodulator*: Regulates and supports immune function
- *Anti-inflammatory*: Reduces inflammation throughout the body
- *Diuretic*: Increases urine production and supports kidney function

Indications:

- Frequent colds, flu, and other infections
- Chronic fatigue and weakness
- Cardiovascular health support
- Adjunct therapy for cancer treatment
- Kidney and liver support

Energetics: Astragalus has a warming and slightly moistening energy. In Traditional Chinese Medicine (TCM), it is believed to tonify the Qi (vital energy) and strengthen the Wei Qi (defensive energy).

Safety and Dosage

Dosage:

- Decoction: 9–30 grams of dried root simmered in water, taken daily
- Tincture: 2–4 mL, taken 3 times daily
- Capsules: 1000–2000 mg, taken 2–3 times daily

Contraindications: Astragalus should be avoided by individuals with autoimmune conditions, as it may stimulate the immune system. It should also be used cautiously in people with diabetes, as it may lower blood sugar levels.

Interactions: Astragalus may interact with immunosuppressant medications, such as those used after organ transplants. It may also enhance the effects of diuretics and hypoglycemic drugs.

Burdock

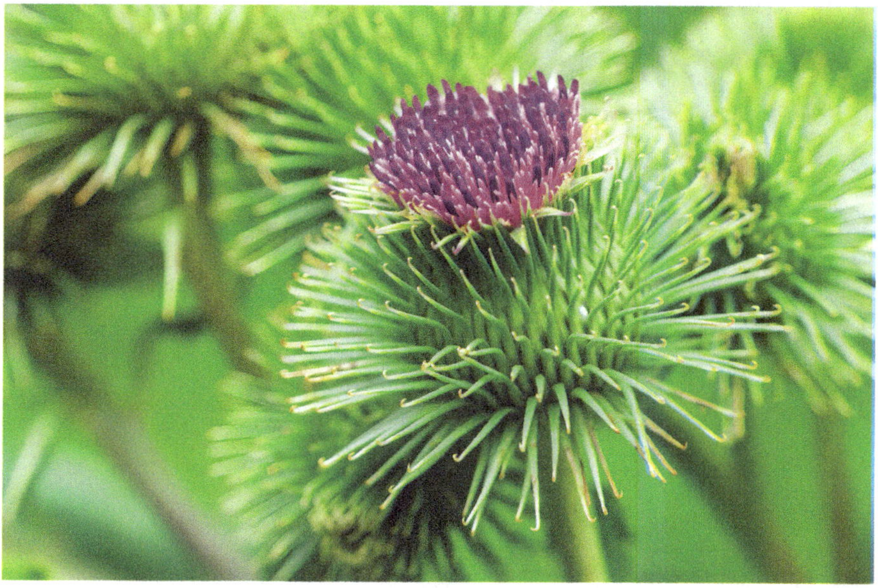

Botanical Information

Scientific Name: *Arctium lappa*

Plant Description: Burdock is a biennial herb that can grow up to two meters tall. It has large, heart-shaped leaves that are dark green and slightly woolly on the underside. The flowers are purple and thistle-like, appearing in the second year of growth. The plant produces round, sticky burrs that easily attach to clothing and animal fur.

Native Region: Burdock is native to Europe and Asia but has been naturalized in many other parts of the world, including North America.

Habitat: This hardy plant can be found growing in disturbed soils, such as along roadsides, in vacant lots, and at the edges of fields and forests. It prefers well-drained, loamy soils and can tolerate partial shade to full sun.

Plant Parts Used: The roots, leaves, and seeds are all used medicinally, with the roots being the most commonly employed part.

Therapeutic Properties

Therapeutic Actions:

- *Alterative*: Supports the body's natural detoxification processes
- *Diuretic*: Increases urine production and supports kidney function
- *Hepatoprotective*: Protects and supports liver function
- *Antibacterial*: Helps fight against bacterial infections
- *Prebiotic*: Promotes the growth of beneficial gut bacteria

Indications:

- Skin conditions, such as acne, eczema, and psoriasis
- Digestive issues, including constipation and indigestion
- Urinary tract infections and kidney stones
- Rheumatic conditions and gout
- Detoxification support

Energetics: Burdock has a cooling and slightly drying energy. It is considered a bitter and sweet herb in Western herbalism.

Safety and Dosage

Dosage:

- Decoction: 2–6 grams of dried root simmered in water, taken 1–3 times daily
- Tincture: 2–4 mL, taken 3 times daily
- Capsules: 1–2 grams of powdered root, taken 3 times daily

Contraindications: Burdock should be used cautiously by individuals with diabetes, as it may lower blood sugar levels. It should also be avoided by people with allergies to plants in the Asteraceae family, such as ragweed and chrysanthemums.

Interactions: Burdock may interact with diuretic and hypoglycemic medications, potentially enhancing their effects. It may also interfere with the absorption of iron and other minerals due to its high tannin content.

Calendula

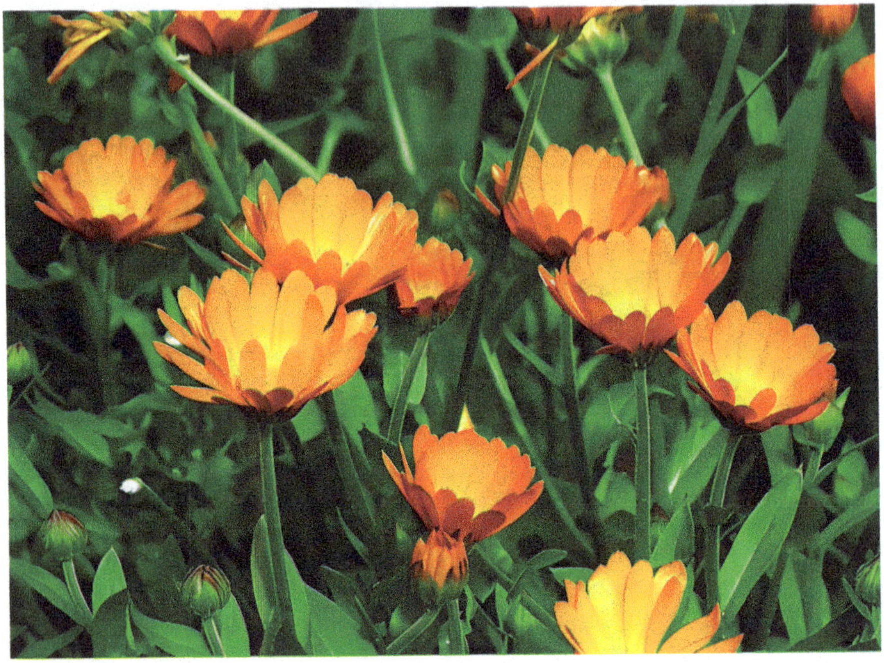

Botanical Information

Scientific Name: *Calendula officinalis*

Plant Description: Calendula, also known as pot marigold, is an annual or short-lived perennial herb that typically grows to a height of 30–60 cm. It has oblong, slightly hairy leaves and produces bright yellow to orange daisy-like flowers. The flowers are composed of numerous tubular and ray florets, giving them a unique, multi-layered appearance.

Native Region: Calendula is native to the Mediterranean region, including southern Europe, northern Africa, and parts of Asia Minor.

Habitat: This adaptable plant thrives in a variety of habitats, including gardens, meadows, and disturbed sites. It prefers well-drained soils and full sun to partial shade.

Plant Parts Used: The flower heads are the primary part used medicinally, often in the form of dried whole flowers or infused oils.

Therapeutic Properties

Therapeutic Actions:

- *Anti-inflammatory:* Reduces inflammation both internally and topically
- *Vulnerary:* Promotes wound healing and tissue repair
- *Antimicrobial:* Helps fight against bacterial and fungal infections
- *Lymphatic:* Stimulates lymphatic drainage and reduces swelling
- *Emmenagogue:* Promotes menstrual flow and regulates the menstrual cycle

Indications:

- Skin conditions, such as cuts, scrapes, burns, and rashes
- Inflammatory digestive issues, including gastritis and ulcers
- Oral health problems, such as gingivitis and mouth ulcers
- Menstrual irregularities and cramps
- Lymphatic congestion and swollen lymph nodes

Energetics: Calendula has a slightly warming and drying energy. It is considered a bitter and pungent herb in Western herbalism.

Safety and Dosage

Dosage:

- Infusion: 1–2 teaspoons of dried flowers per cup of boiling water, steeped for 10–15 minutes, taken 2–3 times daily
- Tincture: 2–4 mL, taken 3 times daily
- Topical: Infused oil or salve applied to the skin as needed

Contraindications: Calendula should be used cautiously by individuals with allergies to plants in the Asteraceae family, such as ragweed and daisies. It should also be avoided during pregnancy, as it may stimulate menstrual flow.

Interactions: Calendula may interact with sedative medications, potentially enhancing their effects. It may also interfere with the body's ability to absorb certain medications due to its high mucilage content.

Chamomile

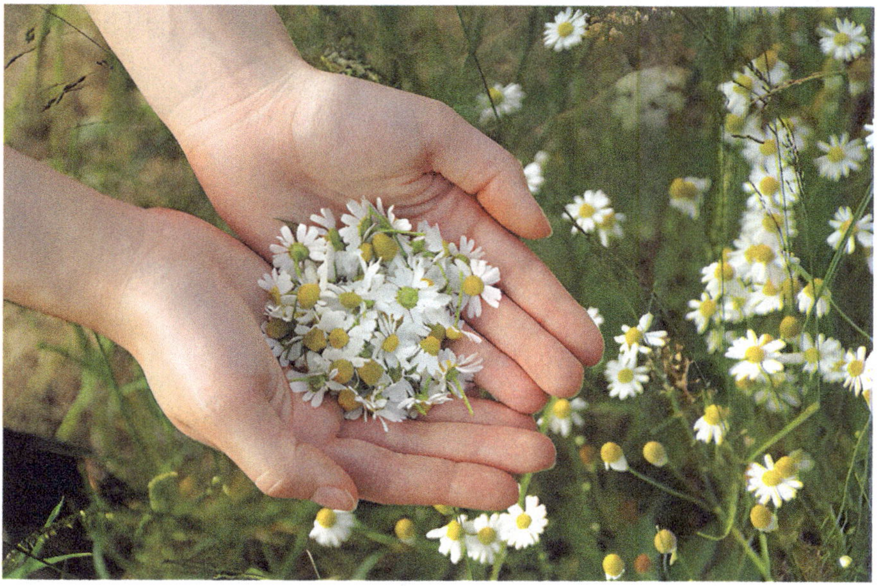

Botanical Information

Scientific Name: *Matricaria chamomilla*

Plant Description: Chamomile is an annual or perennial herb that typically grows to a height of 20–60 cm. It has delicate, bipinnate leaves and produces small, daisy-like flowers with white petals and yellow centers. The flowers have a distinct apple-like aroma and are borne on slender, erect stems.

Native Region: Chamomile is native to Europe and western Asia, but it is now widely cultivated and naturalized in many parts of the world, including North America and Australia.

Habitat: This adaptable plant can be found growing in a variety of habitats, including meadows, pastures, and cultivated fields. It prefers well-drained, sandy, or loamy soils and full sun to partial shade.

Plant Parts Used: The flower heads are the primary part used medicinally, often in the form of dried flowers or essential oil.

Therapeutic Properties

Therapeutic Actions:

- *Anti-inflammatory:* Reduces inflammation both internally and topically
- *Antispasmodic:* Relieves muscle spasms and cramps
- *Carminative:* Helps expel gas and relieve bloating
- *Nervine:* Calms and supports the nervous system
- *Vulnerary:* Promotes wound healing and tissue repair

Indications:

- Digestive issues, such as indigestion, bloating, and cramping
- Anxiety, stress, and insomnia
- Menstrual cramps and PMS symptoms
- Skin inflammation and irritation
- Minor wounds and burns

Energetics: Chamomile has a slightly cooling and drying energy. It is considered a bitter and pungent herb in Western herbalism.

Safety and Dosage

Dosage:

- Infusion: 1–2 teaspoons of dried flowers per cup of boiling water, steeped for 5–10 minutes, taken 3–4 times daily
- Tincture: 1–4 mL, taken 3 times daily
- Essential oil: 1–2 drops in a carrier oil for topical use or inhalation

Contraindications: Chamomile should be used cautiously by individuals with allergies to plants in the Asteraceae family, such as ragweed and daisies. It may also interact with certain medications, such as blood thinners and sedatives.

Interactions: Chamomile may enhance the effects of sedative medications and alcohol. It may also interact with blood-thinning medications, such as warfarin, due to its coumarin content.

Dandelion

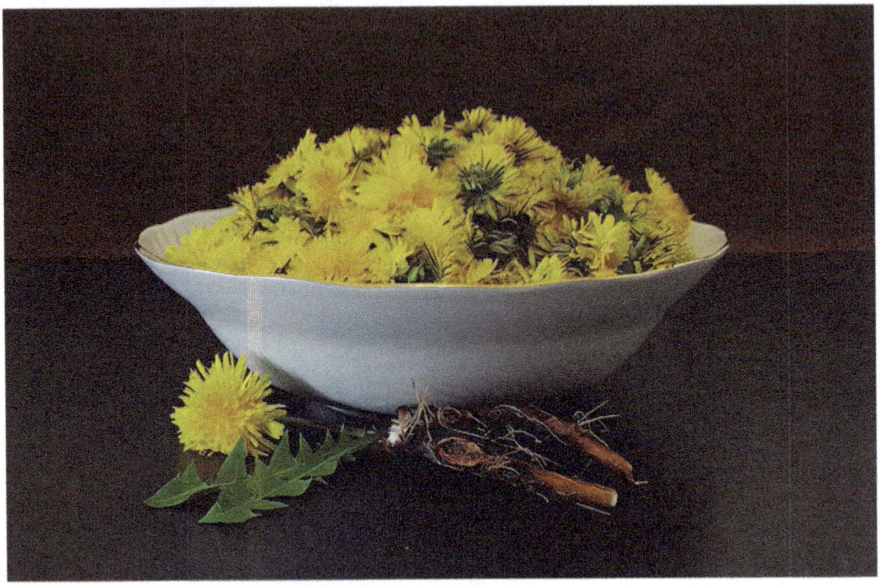

Botanical Information

Scientific Name: *Taraxacum officinale*

Plant Description: Dandelion is a perennial herb that typically grows to a height of 5–40 cm. It has a basal rosette of deeply toothed, lance-shaped leaves and produces bright yellow, composite flowers on hollow stems. The plant exudes a milky white sap when broken and develops a puffball of silver-tufted seeds.

Native Region: Dandelion is native to Europe and Asia but has been naturalized in many parts of the world, including North America, where it is often considered a common weed.

Habitat: This hardy plant can be found growing in a wide variety of habitats, including lawns, meadows, pastures, and disturbed sites. It thrives in full sun and can tolerate a range of soil conditions.

Plant Parts Used: The roots, leaves, and flowers are all used medicinally, each with slightly different therapeutic properties.

Therapeutic Properties

Therapeutic Actions:

- *Cholagogue:* Stimulates bile production and flow
- *Diuretic:* Increases urine production and supports kidney function
- *Bitter tonic:* Stimulates digestion and liver function
- *Prebiotic:* Promotes the growth of beneficial gut bacteria
- *Alterative:* Supports the body's natural detoxification processes

Indications:

- Digestive issues, such as indigestion, bloating, and constipation
- Liver and gallbladder disorders, including non-alcoholic fatty liver disease
- Urinary tract infections and kidney stones
- Skin conditions, such as acne and eczema
- Metabolic disorders, including type 2 diabetes and hyperlipidemia

Energetics: Dandelion has a cooling and drying energy. It is considered a bitter herb in Western herbalism.

Safety and Dosage

Dosage:

- Decoction (roots): 2–4 teaspoons of dried root per cup of water, simmered for 10–15 minutes, taken 3 times daily
- Infusion (leaves): 1–2 teaspoons of dried leaves per cup of boiling water, steeped for 10–15 minutes, taken 3 times daily
- Tincture: 2–5 mL, taken 3 times daily

Contraindications: Dandelion should be used cautiously by individuals with gallstones or bile duct obstruction, as it may stimulate bile flow and exacerbate these conditions. It should also be avoided by people with allergies to plants in the Asteraceae family, such as ragweed and daisies.

Interactions: Dandelion may interact with certain medications, such as diuretics and antibiotics. It may also interfere with the absorption of certain nutrients, such as iron, due to its high tannin content.

Echinacea

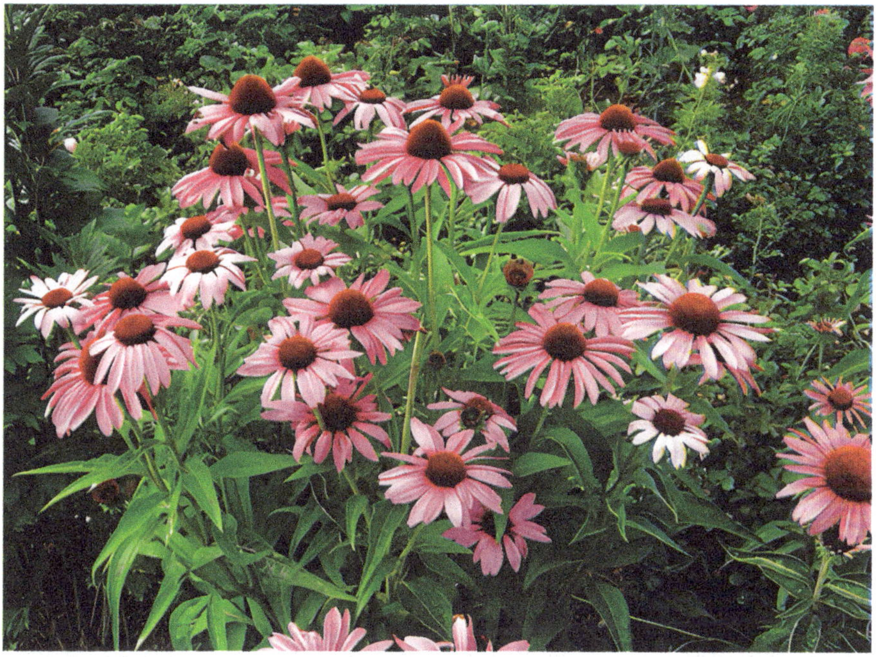

Botanical Information

Scientific Name: *Echinacea purpurea*

Plant Description: Echinacea is a perennial herb that typically grows to a height of 60–180 cm. It has rough, lance-shaped leaves and produces large, showy flowers with purple-pink petals and spiny, cone-shaped centers. The plant has a deep taproot and a fibrous root system.

Native Region: Echinacea is native to the prairies and open woodlands of central and eastern North America, primarily in the United States.

Habitat: This hardy plant thrives in full sun and well-drained soils, often found in prairies, meadows, and open woods. It is drought-tolerant and can adapt to a range of soil conditions.

Plant Parts Used: The roots, leaves, and flowers are all used medicinally, with the roots being the most potent and commonly used part.

Therapeutic Properties

Therapeutic Actions:

- *Immunomodulator:* Regulates and supports immune function
- *Anti-inflammatory:* Reduces inflammation throughout the body
- *Antimicrobial:* Helps fight against bacterial, viral, and fungal infections
- *Lymphatic:* Stimulates lymphatic drainage and reduces swelling
- *Vulnerary:* Promotes wound healing and tissue repair

Indications:

- Acute and chronic infections, such as colds, flu, and respiratory infections
- Immune system disorders, including autoimmune conditions
- Inflammatory conditions, such as arthritis and skin disorders
- Wounds, burns, and other skin injuries
- Lymphatic congestion and swollen lymph nodes

Energetics: Echinacea has a cooling and drying energy. It is considered a pungent and bitter herb in Western herbalism.

Safety and Dosage

Dosage:

- Decoction (roots): 1–2 teaspoons of dried root per cup of water, simmered for 10–15 minutes, taken 3 times daily
- Infusion (leaves/flowers): 1–2 teaspoons of dried herb per cup of boiling water, steeped for 10–15 minutes, taken 3 times daily
- Tincture: 2–4 mL, taken 3 times daily

Contraindications: Echinacea should be used cautiously by individuals with autoimmune conditions, as it may stimulate the immune system and exacerbate symptoms. It should also be avoided by people with allergies to plants in the Asteraceae family, such as ragweed and daisies.

Interactions: Echinacea may interact with certain medications, such as immunosuppressants and chemotherapy drugs. It may also interfere with the body's ability to break down caffeine and certain other drugs metabolized by the liver.

Elderberry

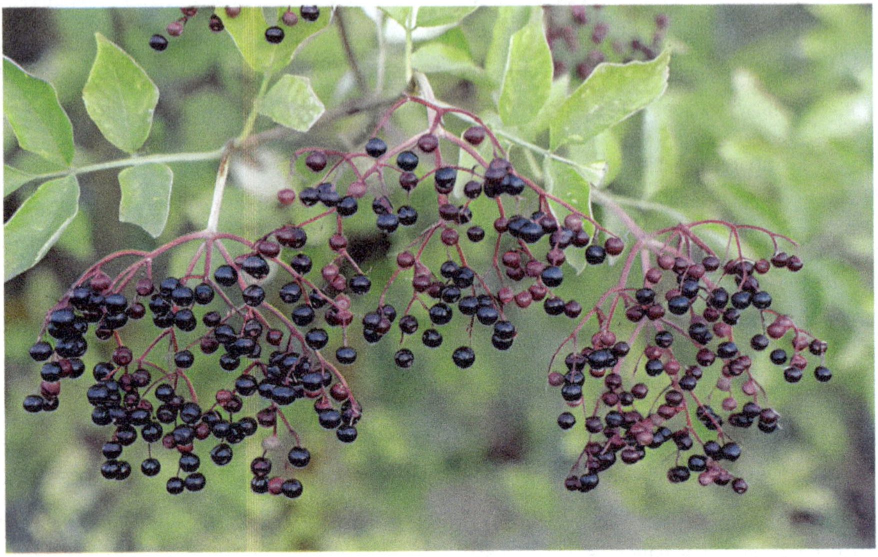

Botanical Information

Scientific Name: Sambucus nigra

Plant Description: Elderberry is a deciduous shrub or small tree that typically grows to a height of 3–6 meters. It has pinnate, compound leaves with 5–7 serrated leaflets and produces large, flat-topped clusters of small, white to cream-colored flowers. The flowers give way to clusters of small, dark purple to black berries.

Native Region: Elderberry is native to Europe, North Africa, and parts of Asia but has been naturalized in many other parts of the world, including North America.

Habitat: This adaptable plant can be found growing in a variety of habitats, including woodlands, hedgerows, and along streams and roadsides. It prefers moist, well-drained soils and can tolerate partial shade to full sun.

Plant Parts Used: The berries and flowers are the primary parts used medicinally, with the berries being more commonly used.

Therapeutic Properties

Therapeutic Actions:

- *Immunomodulator:* Regulates and supports immune function
- *Antiviral:* Helps fight against viral infections, particularly influenza
- *Diaphoretic:* Promotes sweating and helps to lower fever
- *Anti-inflammatory:* Reduces inflammation throughout the body
- *Antioxidant:* Protects cells from damage caused by free radicals

Indications:

- Acute and chronic viral infections, such as colds and flu
- Upper respiratory tract infections, including bronchitis and sinusitis
- Fever and chills
- Inflammatory conditions, such as arthritis and allergies
- General immune system support and disease prevention

Energetics: Elderberry has a cooling and drying energy. It is considered a sweet and slightly bitter herb in Western herbalism.

Safety and Dosage

Dosage:

- Syrup: 1–2 tablespoons, taken 2–3 times daily
- Tincture: 2–4 mL, taken 3 times daily
- Infusion (flowers): 1–2 teaspoons of dried flowers per cup of boiling water, steeped for 10–15 minutes, taken 3 times daily

Contraindications: Elderberry should be used cautiously by individuals with autoimmune conditions, as it may stimulate the immune system and exacerbate symptoms. Raw, unripe berries and other parts of the plant (leaves, bark, roots) contain toxic compounds and should not be consumed.

Interactions: Elderberry may interact with certain medications, such as immunosuppressants and chemotherapy drugs. It may also interfere with the body's ability to break down certain drugs metabolized by the liver.

Fennel

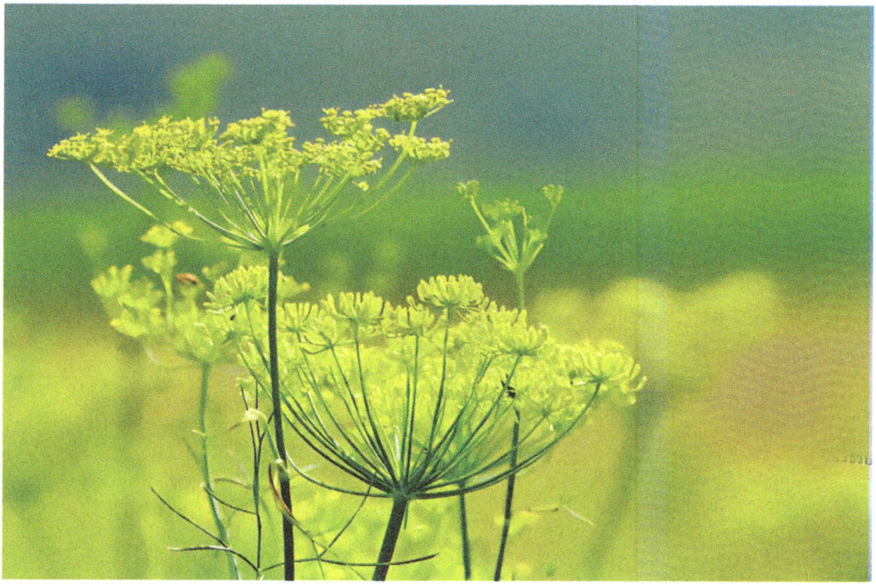

Botanical Information

Scientific Name: *Foeniculum vulgare*

Plant Description: Fennel is an aromatic, perennial herb that typically grows to a height of 1–2 meters. It has finely divided, feathery leaves and produces umbels of small, yellow flowers. The plant has a thick, fleshy taproot and a hollow, ridged stem with a distinctive anise-like aroma.

Native Region: Fennel is native to the Mediterranean region but has been naturalized in many other parts of the world, including Asia, Europe, and North America.

Habitat: This hardy plant thrives in full sun and well-drained soils, often found growing in fields, along roadsides, and in cultivated gardens. It is drought-tolerant and can adapt to a range of soil conditions.

Plant Parts Used: The seeds, leaves, and bulb are all used medicinally and as culinary herbs, each with slightly different therapeutic properties.

Therapeutic Properties

Therapeutic Actions:

- *Carminative:* Helps expel gas and relieve bloating
- *Digestive:* Stimulates digestion and supports overall digestive function
- *Galactagogue*: Promotes lactation in nursing mothers
- *Expectorant:* Helps to expel mucus from the lungs and airways
- *Antispasmodic:* Relieves muscle spasms and cramping

Indications:

- Digestive issues, such as bloating, gas, and indigestion
- Respiratory conditions, including bronchitis and coughs
- Menstrual cramps and PMS symptoms
- Insufficient milk production in nursing mothers
- Stress and anxiety-related digestive disturbances

Energetics: Fennel has a slightly warming and drying energy. It is considered a sweet and pungent herb in Western herbalism.

Safety and Dosage

Dosage:

- Infusion (seeds): 1–2 teaspoons of crushed seeds per cup of boiling water, steeped for 10-15 minutes, taken 2–3 times daily
- Tincture: 1–2 mL, taken 2–3 times daily
- Capsules: 1–2 capsules (500 mg–1 g), taken 2–3 times daily

Contraindications: Fennel should be used cautiously by individuals with estrogen-sensitive conditions, such as breast or ovarian cancer, as it may have mild estrogenic effects. Large doses may cause photosensitivity in some individuals.

Interactions: Fennel may interact with certain medications, such as birth control pills and hormone replacement therapies, due to its potential estrogenic effects. It may also interfere with the absorption of certain antibiotics and other medications.

Ginger

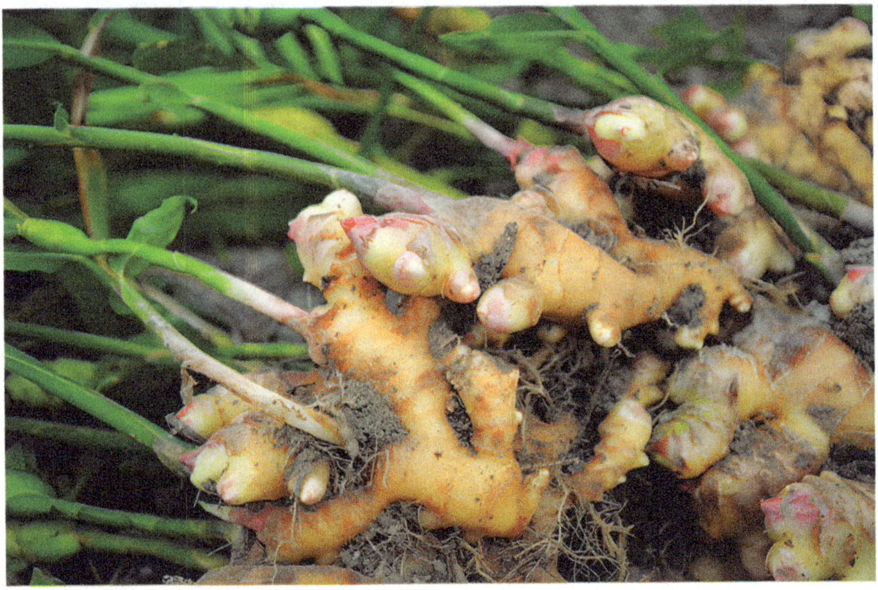

Botanical Information

Scientific Name: *Zingiber officinale*

Plant Description: Ginger is a perennial, herbaceous plant that typically grows to a height of 30–100 cm. It has long, lanceolate leaves and produces clusters of white or yellow flowers. The plant has a thick, knotted rhizome that grows horizontally just beneath the soil surface.

Native Region: Ginger is native to Southeast Asia, particularly India and China, but is now cultivated in many tropical and subtropical regions worldwide.

Habitat: This tropical plant thrives in warm, humid climates with partial shade and rich, well-drained soils. It is often grown as a cash crop in tropical countries.

Plant Parts Used: The rhizome, or underground stem, is the primary part used medicinally and as a culinary spice.

Therapeutic Properties

Therapeutic Actions:

- *Carminative:* Helps expel gas and relieve bloating
- *Anti-inflammatory:* Reduces inflammation throughout the body
- *Antiemetic:* Helps to relieve nausea and vomiting
- *Analgesic:* Provides pain relief, particularly for muscle and joint pain
- *Circulatory stimulant:* Improves blood flow and warms the body

Indications:

- Digestive issues, such as indigestion, bloating, and gas
- Nausea and vomiting, including motion sickness and morning sickness
- Inflammatory conditions, such as arthritis and muscle soreness
- Menstrual cramps and PMS symptoms
- Respiratory conditions, including colds, flu, and bronchitis

Energetics: Ginger has a warming and slightly drying energy. It is considered a pungent and spicy herb in Western herbalism.

Safety and Dosage

Dosage:

- Infusion: 1–2 teaspoons of grated fresh rhizome or 1/2–1 teaspoon of dried powder per cup of boiling water, steeped for 10–15 minutes, taken 2–3 times daily
- Tincture: 1–2 mL, taken 2–3 times daily
- Capsules: 1–2 capsules (500 mg–1 g), taken 2–3 times daily

Contraindications: Ginger should be used cautiously by individuals with gallstones, as it may stimulate the release of bile. Large doses may cause heartburn or other gastrointestinal discomfort in some individuals.

Interactions: Ginger may interact with certain medications, such as blood thinners and diabetes medications, due to its blood-thinning and hypoglycemic effects. It may also interfere with the absorption of some medications, such as cyclosporine.

Goldenseal

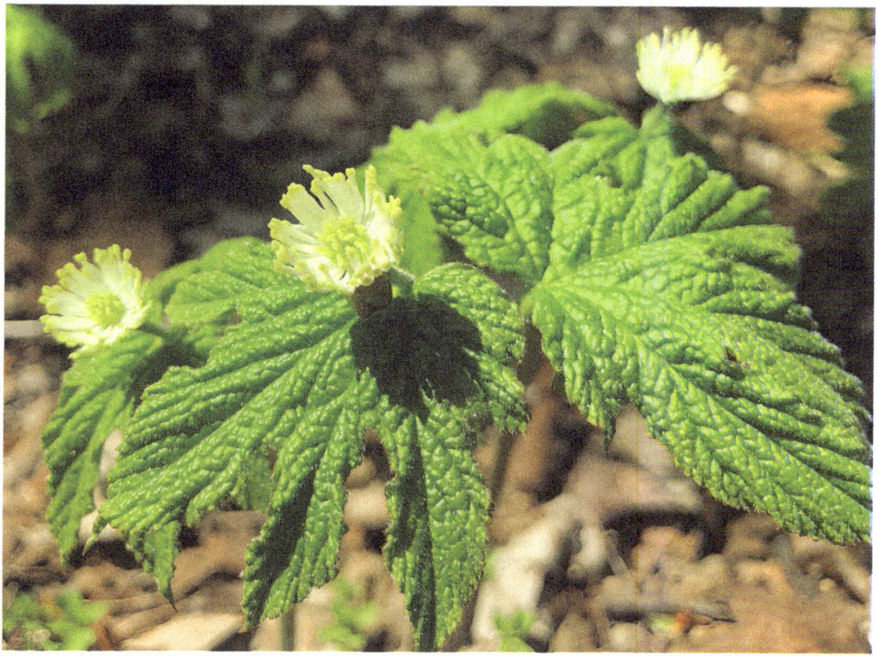

Botanical Information

Scientific Name: *Hydrastis canadensis*

Plant Description: Goldenseal is a perennial herb that typically grows to a height of 20–50 cm. It has a thick, yellow rhizome that gives rise to a single stem with two palmate, lobed leaves. The plant produces a solitary, greenish-white flower that develops into a raspberry-like fruit.

Native Region: Goldenseal is native to the hardwood forests of eastern North America, primarily in the United States and Canada.

Habitat: This woodland plant thrives in rich, moist soils under the dappled shade of deciduous trees. It is often found growing in small patches in the understory of mature forests.

Plant Parts Used: The rhizome and roots are the primary parts used medicinally, often in dried or powdered form.

Therapeutic Properties

Therapeutic Actions:

- *Antimicrobial:* Helps fight against bacterial, viral, and fungal infections
- *Anti-inflammatory:* Reduces inflammation throughout the body
- *Astringent:* Tightens and tones tissues, particularly mucous membranes
- *Bitter tonic:* Stimulates digestion and liver function
- *Immune stimulant:* Enhances immune system activity

Indications:

- Digestive issues, such as peptic ulcers and inflammatory bowel disease
- Upper respiratory tract infections, including sinusitis and bronchitis
- Urinary tract infections and cystitis
- Skin infections and wounds
- Oral health issues, such as gingivitis and canker sores

Energetics: Goldenseal has a cooling and drying energy. It is considered a bitter and astringent herb in Western herbalism.

Safety and Dosage

Dosage:

- Decoction: 1/2–1 teaspoon of dried rhizome per cup of water, simmered for 10–15 minutes, taken 2–3 times daily
- Tincture: 1–2 mL, taken 2–3 times daily
- Capsules: 1–2 capsules (500 mg–1 g), taken 2–3 times daily

Contraindications: Goldenseal should not be used during pregnancy, as it may stimulate uterine contractions. It should also be avoided by individuals with high blood pressure or heart conditions, as it may raise blood pressure.

Interactions: Goldenseal may interact with certain medications, such as antibiotics and blood pressure medications. It may also interfere with the absorption of B vitamins and other nutrients.

Holy Basil

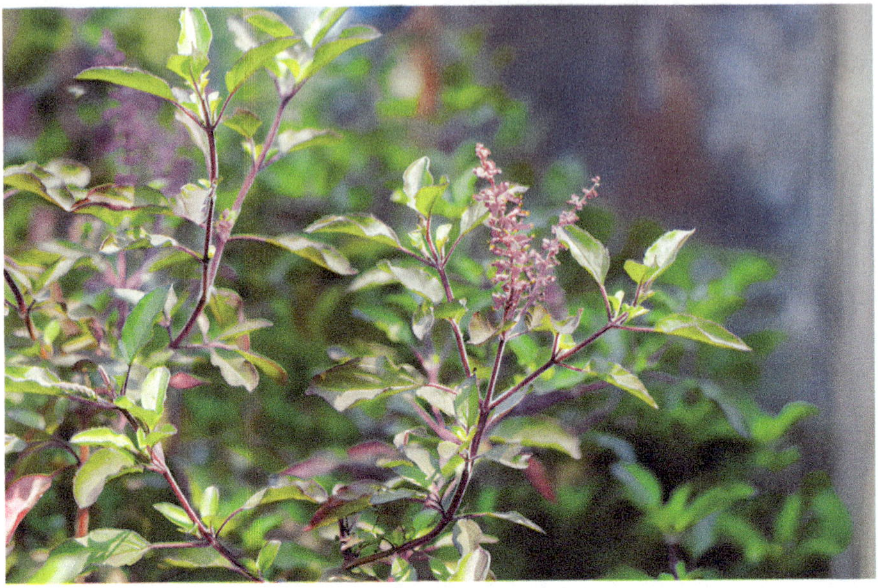

Botanical Information

Scientific Name: *Ocimum sanctum*

Plant Description: Holy Basil, also known as Tulsi, is a perennial herb that typically grows to a height of 30–60 cm. It has a woody stem that gives rise to many branches with opposite, ovate leaves. The plant produces small, purple, or white flowers arranged in whorls on spikes.

Native Region: Holy Basil is native to the Indian subcontinent and is widely cultivated throughout Southeast Asia.

Habitat: This adaptable plant can grow in a variety of habitats, from moist, fertile soils to dry, rocky areas. It is often cultivated in home gardens and near Hindu temples.

Plant Parts Used: The leaves and flowering tops are the primary parts used medicinally, often in fresh or dried form.

Therapeutic Properties

Therapeutic Actions:

- *Adaptogen:* Helps the body adapt to stress and promotes homeostasis
- *Immunomodulator:* Regulates and supports immune function
- *Anti-inflammatory:* Reduces inflammation throughout the body
- *Antioxidant:* Protects cells from damage caused by free radicals
- *Nootropic:* Enhances cognitive function and memory

Indications:

- Stress, anxiety, and depression
- Respiratory conditions, such as bronchitis and asthma
- Digestive issues, including bloating and indigestion
- Metabolic disorders, such as diabetes and hyperlipidemia
- Cognitive decline and memory impairment

Energetics: Holy Basil has a warming and slightly drying energy. It is considered a pungent and bitter herb in Ayurvedic medicine.

Safety and Dosage

Dosage:

- Infusion: 1–2 teaspoons of dried herb per cup of boiling water, steeped for 10–15 minutes, taken 2–3 times daily
- Tincture: 2–4 mL, taken 2–3 times daily
- Capsules: 1–2 capsules (500 mg–1 g), taken 2–3 times daily

Contraindications: Holy Basil should be used cautiously by individuals with low blood sugar, as it may further reduce glucose levels. It may also interact with medications metabolized by the liver.

Interactions: Holy Basil may interact with certain medications, such as blood thinners and diabetes medications. It may also potentiate the effects of sedatives and CNS depressants.

Hops

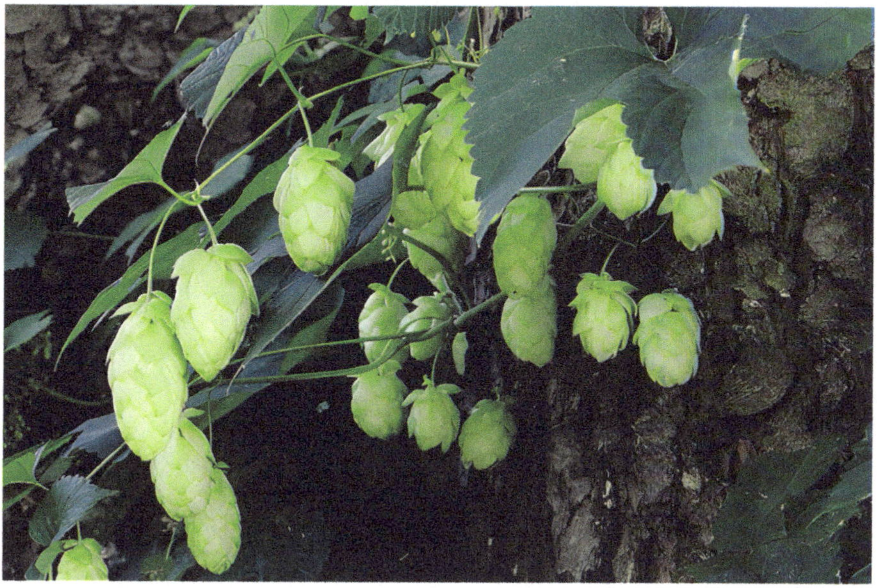

Botanical Information

Scientific Name: *Humulus lupulus*

Plant Description: Hops is a perennial, climbing vine that can grow up to 6–9 meters in length. It has opposite, lobed leaves and produces cone-like female flowers that are used in brewing and herbal medicine. The plant has a thick, branching rhizome that gives rise to many bine-like stems.

Native Region: Hops is native to Europe, western Asia, and North America but is now cultivated worldwide, primarily for its use in the brewing industry.

Habitat: This adaptable plant can grow in a variety of habitats, from moist, fertile soils to dry, rocky areas. It is often cultivated in large, trellised fields known as "hop yards."

Plant Parts Used: The female flowering cones, also known as "Strobiles," are the primary parts used medicinally and in brewing. The young shoots, called hop sprouts, are also eaten as a vegetable.

Therapeutic Properties

Therapeutic Actions:

- *Sedative:* Promotes relaxation and aids in sleep
- *Anxiolytic:* Helps to relieve anxiety and nervousness
- *Bitter tonic:* Stimulates digestion and liver function
- *Estrogenic:* Contains phytoestrogens that can mimic the effects of estrogen in the body
- *Antimicrobial:* Helps fight against bacterial and fungal infections

Indications:

- Insomnia and sleep disorders
- Anxiety and nervous tension
- Digestive issues, such as indigestion and dyspepsia
- Menopausal symptoms, including hot flashes and mood swings
- Skin conditions, such as eczema and dermatitis

Energetics: Hops has a cooling and drying energy. It is considered a bitter and pungent herb in Western herbalism.

Safety and Dosage

Dosage:

- Infusion: 1–2 teaspoons of dried Strobiles per cup of boiling water, steeped for 10–15 minutes, taken 2–3 times daily
- Tincture: 1–2 mL, taken 2–3 times daily
- Capsules: 1–2 capsules (500 mg–1 g), taken 2–3 times daily

Contraindications: Hops should be used cautiously by individuals with depression, as it may exacerbate symptoms. It should also be avoided by pregnant women, as it may stimulate uterine contractions.

Interactions: Hops may interact with certain medications, such as sedatives and sleep aids, potentially enhancing their effects. It may also interfere with the absorption of iron and other minerals.

Lavender

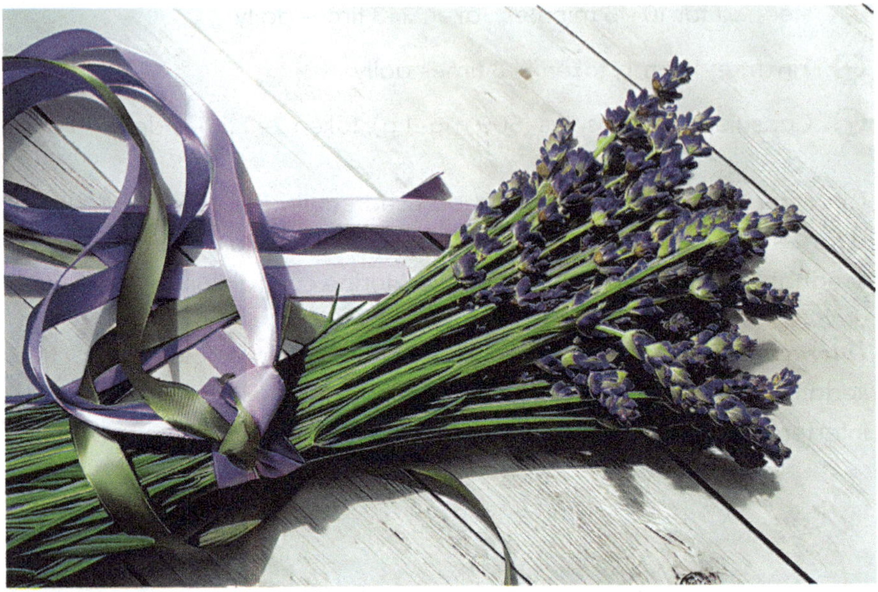

Botanical Information

Scientific Name: *Lavandula angustifolia*

Plant Description: Lavender is a perennial, evergreen shrub that typically grows to a height of 30–60 cm. It has woody stems that give rise to linear, gray-green leaves and produce spikes of small, purple flowers. The plant has a strong, distinctive aroma that is prized in perfumery and herbal medicine.

Native Region: Lavender is native to the Mediterranean region, including southern Europe, northern Africa, and parts of the Middle East.

Habitat: This hardy plant thrives in sunny, well-drained soils and can tolerate drought and heat. It is often grown in large, cultivated fields known as "lavender farms."

Plant Parts Used: The flowers are the primary parts used medicinally and in aromatherapy. The leaves and essential oils are also used in some applications.

Therapeutic Properties

Therapeutic Actions:

- *Anxiolytic*: Helps to relieve anxiety and nervousness
- *Sedative:* Promotes relaxation and aids in sleep
- *Carminative:* Helps expel gas and relieve bloating
- *Antimicrobial:* Helps fight against bacterial and fungal infections
- *Analgesic:* Provides pain relief, particularly for headaches and muscle tension

Indications:

- Anxiety and stress-related disorders
- Insomnia and sleep disturbances
- Digestive issues, such as bloating and indigestion
- Headaches and migraines
- Skin conditions, such as acne and eczema

Energetics: Lavender has a cooling and slightly drying energy. It is considered a pungent and slightly bitter herb in Western herbalism.

Safety and Dosage

Dosage:

- Infusion: 1–2 teaspoons of dried flowers per cup of boiling water, steeped for 10–15 minutes, taken 2–3 times daily
- Tincture: 1–2 mL, taken 2–3 times daily

- Essential oil: 1–2 drops diluted in a carrier oil for topical application or inhalation

Contraindications: Lavender is generally considered safe for most individuals. However, it may cause allergic reactions in some people, particularly those with sensitivities to other plants in the Lamiaceae family.

Interactions: Lavender may interact with certain medications, such as sedatives and sleep aids, potentially enhancing their effects. It may also interfere with the absorption of iron and other minerals.

Lemon Balm

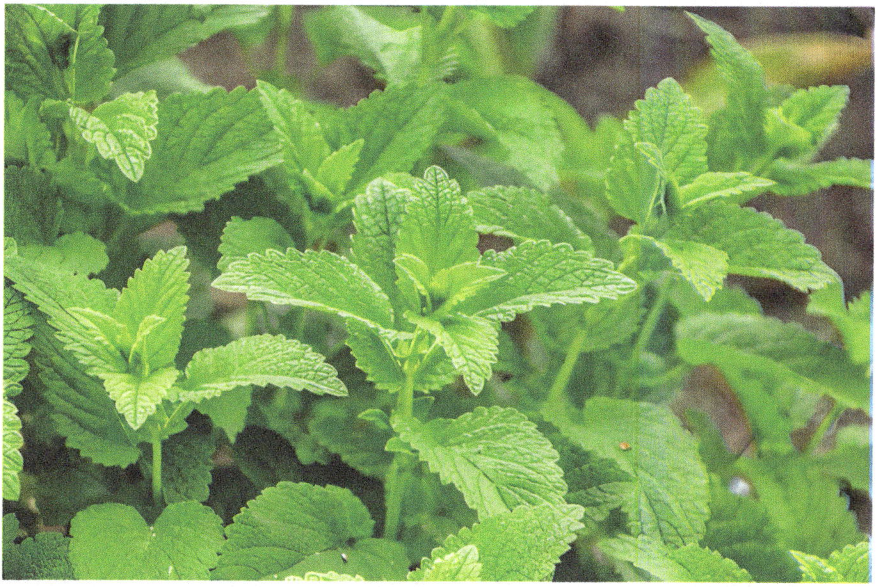

Botanical Information

Scientific Name: *Melissa officinalis*

Plant Description: Lemon Balm is a perennial herb that typically grows to a height of 30–90 cm. It has a square stem that gives rise to opposite, ovate leaves with serrated edges. The plant produces small, white, or yellowish flowers that appear in loose clusters.

Native Region: Lemon Balm is native to the Mediterranean region, including southern Europe, northern Africa, and parts of the Middle East.

Habitat: This adaptable plant can grow in a variety of habitats, from moist, fertile soils to dry, rocky areas. It is often cultivated in herb gardens and can naturalize in temperate regions.

Plant Parts Used: The leaves are the primary parts used medicinally, often in fresh or dried form. The essential oil is also used in aromatherapy and skincare products.

Therapeutic Properties

Therapeutic Actions:

- *Anxiolytic*: Helps to relieve anxiety and nervousness
- *Sedative*: Promotes relaxation and aids in sleep
- *Carminative*: Helps expel gas and relieve bloating
- *Antiviral*: Helps fight against viral infections, particularly herpes simplex virus
- *Nootropic*: Enhances cognitive function and memory

Indications:

- Anxiety and stress-related disorders
- Insomnia and sleep disturbances
- Digestive issues, such as bloating and indigestion
- Viral infections, including cold sores and herpes
- Cognitive decline and memory impairment

Energetics: Lemon Balm has a cooling and slightly drying energy. It is considered a pungent and slightly bitter herb in Western herbalism.

Safety and Dosage

Dosage:

- Infusion: 1–2 teaspoons of dried herb per cup of boiling water, steeped for 10–15 minutes, taken 2–3 times daily
- Tincture: 2–4 mL, taken 2–3 times daily
- Capsules: 1–2 capsules (500 mg–1 g), taken 2–3 times daily

Contraindications: Lemon Balm is generally considered safe for most individuals. However, it may cause drowsiness in some people and should be used cautiously by those operating heavy machinery or driving.

Interactions: Lemon Balm may interact with certain medications, such as sedatives and thyroid medications. It may also interfere with the absorption of iron and other minerals.

Licorice

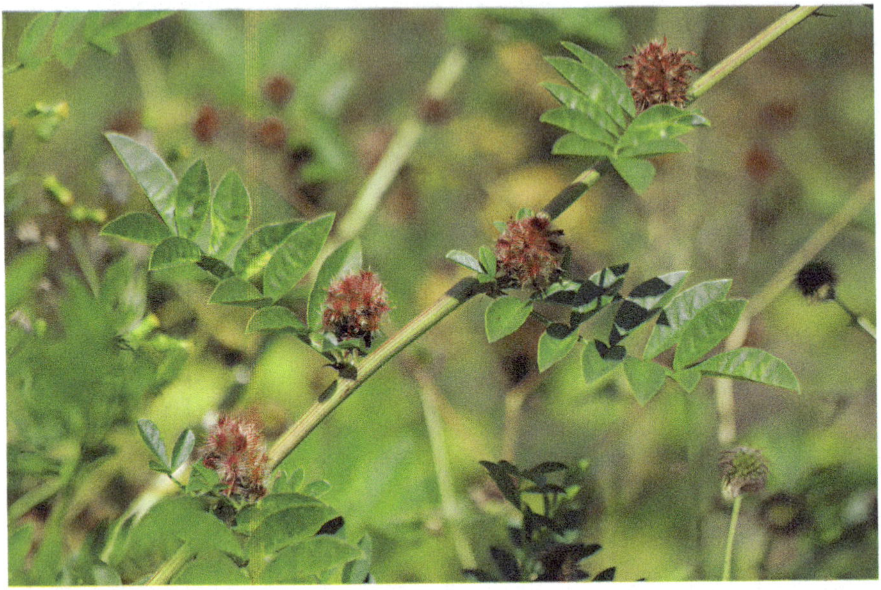

Botanical Information

Scientific Name: *Glycyrrhiza glabra*

Plant Description: Licorice is a perennial herb that typically grows to a height of 1–2 meters. It has pinnate, compound leaves and produces spikes of pale blue or violet flowers. The plant has an extensive root system that can reach depths of up to 1 meter.

Native Region: Licorice is native to the Mediterranean region, including southern Europe, northern Africa, and parts of the Middle East.

Habitat: This hardy plant can grow in a variety of habitats, from moist, fertile soils to dry, sandy areas. It is often cultivated in large fields for commercial use.

Plant Parts Used: The roots and rhizomes are the primary parts used medicinally, often in dried or powdered form. The leaves are also used in some traditional medicine systems.

Therapeutic Properties

Therapeutic Actions:

- *Demulcent*: Soothes and protects mucous membranes
- *Expectorant*: Helps to expel mucus from the lungs and airways
- *Adaptogen*: Helps the body adapt to stress and promotes homeostasis
- *Anti-inflammatory*: Reduces inflammation throughout the body
- *Antiviral*: Helps fight against viral infections, particularly hepatitis and HIV

Indications:

- Digestive issues, such as ulcers and gastritis
- Respiratory conditions, including bronchitis and asthma
- Adrenal fatigue and chronic stress
- Inflammatory conditions, such as arthritis and eczema
- Viral infections, including hepatitis and HIV

Energetics: Licorice has a warming and moistening energy. It is considered a sweet and slightly bitter herb in Western herbalism.

Safety and Dosage

Dosage:

- Decoction: 1–2 teaspoons of dried root per cup of water, simmered for 10–15 minutes, taken 2–3 times daily
- Tincture: 1–2 mL, taken 2–3 times daily
- Capsules: 1–2 capsules (500 mg–1 g), taken 2–3 times daily

Contraindications: Licorice should be used cautiously by individuals with hypertension, as it can raise blood pressure in high doses. It should also be avoided by pregnant women, as it may increase the risk of preterm labor.

Interactions: Licorice may interact with certain medications, such as diuretics, corticosteroids, and blood thinners. It may also interfere with the body's potassium levels and should be used cautiously by those with kidney disorders.

Nettle

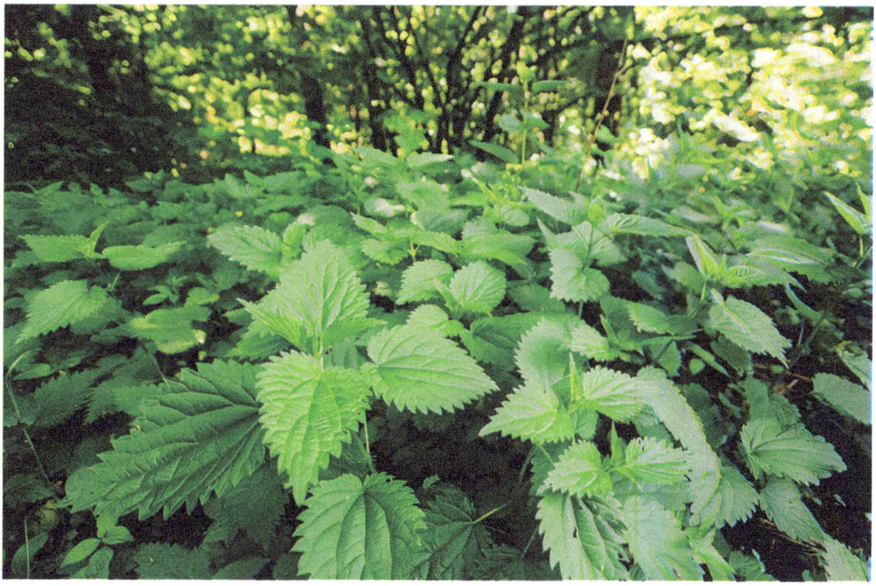

Botanical Information

Scientific Name: *Urtica dioica*

Plant Description: Nettle is a perennial herb that typically grows to a height of 1–2 meters. It has opposite, heart-shaped leaves with serrated edges and is covered in stinging hairs that can cause a painful rash upon contact. The plant produces small, greenish flowers that appear in clusters.

Native Region: Nettle is native to Europe, Asia, and parts of North Africa but has been naturalized in many other parts of the world, including North America.

Habitat: This adaptable plant can grow in a variety of habitats, from moist, fertile soils to dry, rocky areas. It is often found in disturbed areas, such as along roadsides and in abandoned fields.

Plant Parts Used: The leaves and roots are the primary parts used medicinally, often in dried or powdered form. The young shoots are also eaten as a nutritious vegetable.

Therapeutic Properties

Therapeutic Actions:

- *Diuretic:* Increases urine production and supports kidney function
- *Nutritive:* Provides a wide range of vitamins and minerals, including iron and calcium
- *Anti-inflammatory:* Reduces inflammation throughout the body
- *Astringent:* Tightens and tones tissues, particularly in the urinary tract
- *Galactagogue:* Promotes lactation in nursing mothers

Indications:

- Urinary tract infections and kidney stones
- Anemia and other nutritional deficiencies
- Allergies and hay fever
- Arthritis and other inflammatory conditions
- Insufficient milk production in nursing mothers

Energetics: Nettle has a cooling and drying energy. It is considered a pungent and slightly bitter herb in Western herbalism.

Safety and Dosage

Dosage:

- Infusion: 1–2 teaspoons of dried herb per cup of boiling water, steeped for 10–15 minutes, taken 2–3 times daily
- Tincture: 2–4 mL, taken 2–3 times daily
- Capsules: 1–2 capsules (500 mg–1 g), taken 2–3 times daily

Contraindications: Nettle should be used cautiously by individuals with diabetes, as it may lower blood sugar levels. It should also be avoided by those taking blood thinners, as it may increase the risk of bleeding.

Interactions: Nettle may interact with certain medications, such as diuretics, blood thinners, and diabetes medications. It may also interfere with the absorption of iron and other minerals.

Passionflower

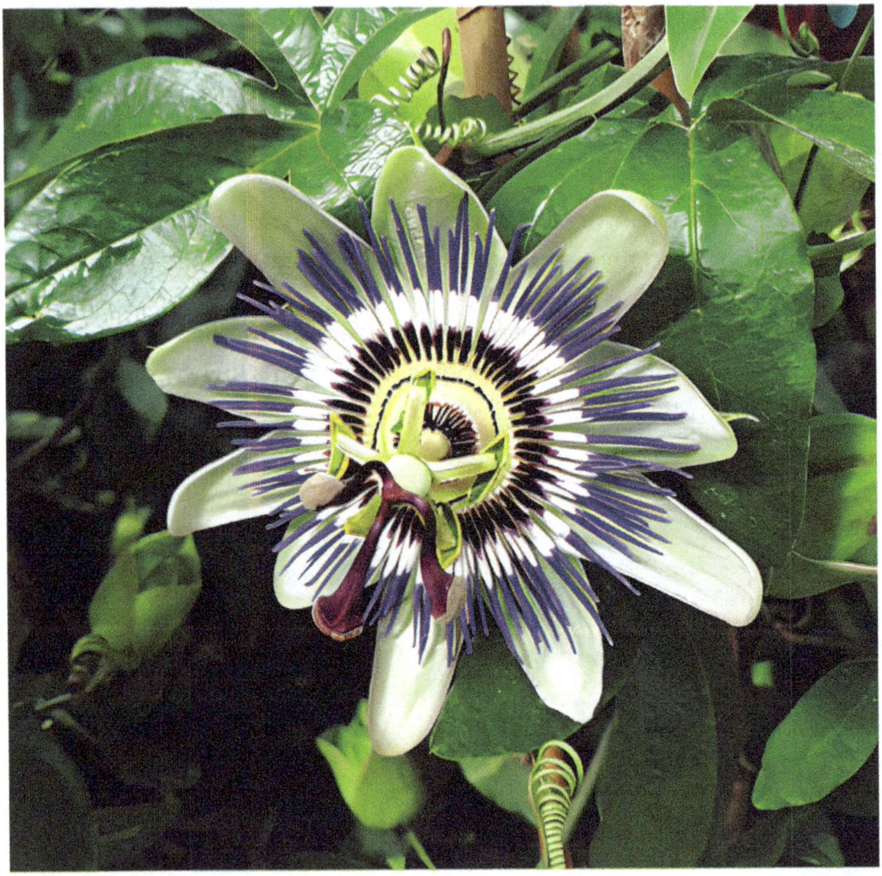

Botanical Information

Scientific Name: *Passiflora incarnata*

Plant Description: Passionflower is a perennial, climbing vine that can grow up to 9 meters in length. It has alternate, palmate leaves and produces showy, complex flowers with purple and white petals. The plant bears an egg-shaped, edible fruit known as a maypop.

Native Region: Passionflower is native to the southeastern United States, from Virginia to Florida and west to Texas and Oklahoma.

Habitat: This climbing vine typically grows in sunny, disturbed areas such as roadsides, fence rows, and forest edges. It prefers well-drained, sandy or loamy soils.

Plant Parts Used: The aerial parts (leaves, stems, and flowers) are the primary parts used medicinally, often in dried form. The fruits are also edible and are sometimes used in culinary applications.

Therapeutic Properties

Therapeutic Actions:

- *Anxiolytic:* Helps to relieve anxiety and nervousness
- *Sedative:* Promotes relaxation and aids in sleep
- *Antispasmodic:* Relieves muscle spasms and tension
- *Anodyne:* Provides pain relief, particularly for menstrual cramps and headaches
- *Hypotensive:* May help to lower blood pressure

Indications:

- Anxiety and stress-related disorders
- Insomnia and sleep disturbances
- Muscle tension and spasms
- Menstrual cramps and PMS symptoms
- Hypertension and palpitations

Energetics: Passionflower has a cooling and slightly drying energy. It is considered a bitter and pungent herb in Western herbalism.

Safety and Dosage

Dosage:

- Infusion: 1–2 teaspoons of dried herb per cup of boiling water, steeped for 10–15 minutes, taken 2–3 times daily
- Tincture: 2–4 mL, taken 2–3 times daily
- Capsules: 1–2 capsules (500 mg–1 g), taken 2–3 times daily

Contraindications: Passionflower should be used cautiously by pregnant women, as it may stimulate uterine contractions. It should also be avoided by individuals taking sedative medications, as it may enhance their effects.

Interactions: Passionflower may interact with certain medications, such as sedatives, antianxiety drugs, and blood pressure medications. It may also interfere with the absorption of iron and other minerals.

Peppermint

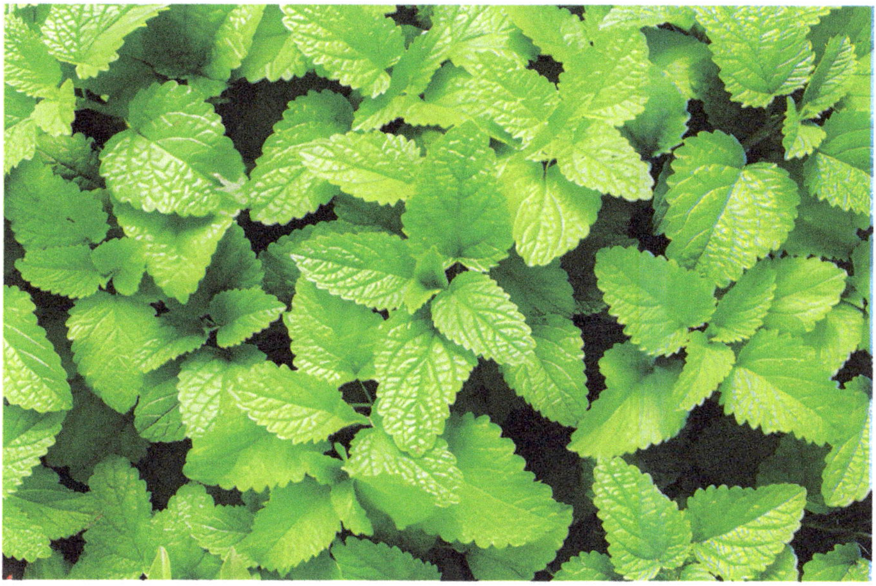

Botanical Information

Scientific Name: *Mentha x piperita*

Plant Description: Peppermint is a perennial herb that typically grows to a height of 30–90 cm. It has square stems that give rise to opposite, ovate leaves with serrated edges. The plant produces small, purple flowers that appear in whorls on terminal spikes.

Native Region: Peppermint is a hybrid species that is believed to have originated in England in the 17th century. It is now widely cultivated throughout Europe, North America, and other temperate regions.

Habitat: This hardy plant can grow in a variety of habitats but prefers moist, rich soils and partial shade. It is often cultivated in large fields for commercial use.

Plant Parts Used: The leaves and essential oil are the primary parts used medicinally. The leaves are often used in dried or fresh form, while the oil is used in aromatherapy, topical applications, and flavoring.

Therapeutic Properties

Therapeutic Actions:

- *Carminative*: Helps expel gas and relieve bloating
- *Analgesic*: Provides pain relief, particularly for headaches and muscle tension
- *Antispasmodic*: Relieves muscle spasms and cramps
- *Antimicrobial*: Helps fight against bacterial and fungal infections
- *Nervine*: Calms and supports the nervous system

Indications:

- Digestive issues, such as indigestion, bloating, and IBS
- Headaches and migraines
- Muscle aches and pains
- Respiratory infections and congestion
- Stress and anxiety

Energetics: Peppermint has a cooling and slightly drying energy. It is considered a pungent and slightly bitter herb in Western herbalism.

Safety and Dosage

Dosage:

- Infusion: 1–2 teaspoons of dried herb per cup of boiling water, steeped for 10–15 minutes, taken 2–3 times daily
- Tincture: 1–2 mL, taken 2–3 times daily

- Essential oil: 1–2 drops diluted in a carrier oil for topical application or inhalation

Contraindications: Peppermint should be used cautiously by individuals with GERD or hiatal hernias, as it may exacerbate symptoms. It should also be avoided by those taking cyclosporine, as it may increase the drug's side effects.

Interactions: Peppermint may interact with certain medications, such as calcium channel blockers and cyclosporine. It may also interfere with the absorption of iron and other minerals.

Rhodiola

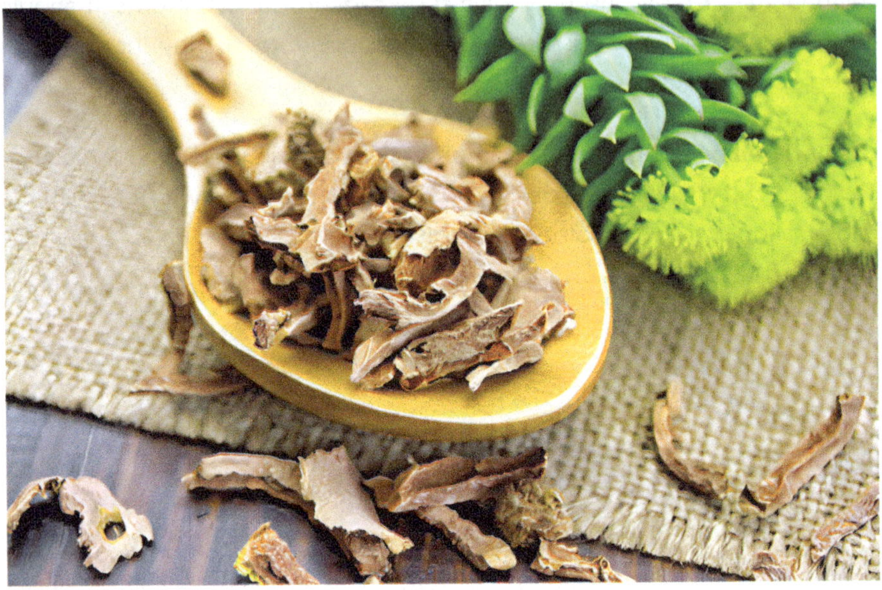

Botanical Information

Scientific Name: *Rhodiola rosea*

Plant Description: Rhodiola is a perennial herb that typically grows to a height of 10–30 cm. It has thick, succulent leaves and produces small, yellow flowers in terminal clusters. The plant has a thick, fragrant rhizome that is often red or golden in color.

Native Region: Rhodiola is native to the Arctic regions of Europe, Asia, and North America, including parts of Siberia, Scandinavia, and Alaska.

Habitat: This hardy plant grows in cold, mountainous regions, often in rocky or sandy soils. It can be found at high altitudes, up to 2,280 meters above sea level.

Plant Parts Used: The rhizome and roots are the primary parts used medicinally, often in dried or powdered form.

Therapeutic Properties

Therapeutic Actions:

- *Adaptogen:* Helps the body adapt to stress and promotes homeostasis
- *Nervine:* Calms and supports the nervous system
- *Nootropic:* Enhances cognitive function and memory
- *Antidepressant:* May help alleviate symptoms of depression
- *Cardioprotective:* Supports cardiovascular health and function

Indications:

- Stress and burnout
- Fatigue and weakness
- Anxiety and depression
- Cognitive decline and memory impairment
- Cardiovascular disorders

Energetics: Rhodiola has a warming and slightly drying energy. It is considered a sweet and slightly bitter herb in Western herbalism.

Safety and Dosage

Dosage:

- Decoction: 1–2 teaspoons of dried rhizome per cup of water, simmered for 10–15 minutes, taken 2–3 times daily
- Tincture: 2–3 mL, taken 2–3 times daily
- Capsules: 1–2 capsules (200–600 mg), taken 1–2 times daily

Contraindications: Rhodiola should be used cautiously by individuals with bipolar disorder, as it may potentially trigger mania. It should also be avoided by those taking MAO inhibitors, as it may interact with these medications.

Interactions: Rhodiola may interact with certain medications, such as antidepressants, anxiolytics, and hormonal medications. It may also potentiate the effects of stimulants, such as caffeine.

Rosemary

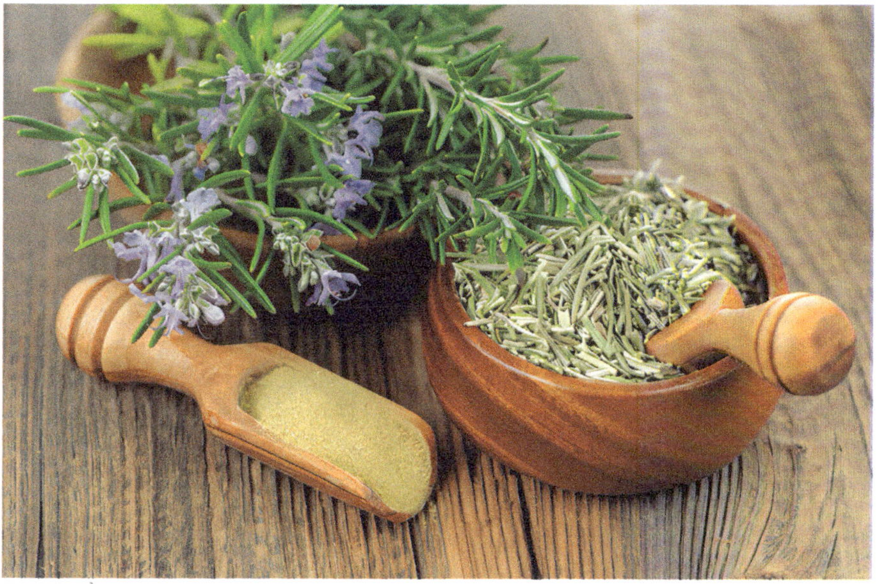

Botanical Information

Scientific Name: *Salvia rosmarinus*

Plant Description: Rosemary is an evergreen shrub that typically grows to a height of 1–2 meters. It has linear, needle-like leaves and produces small, pale blue flowers in clusters along the stems. The plant has a strong, resinous aroma.

Native Region: Rosemary is native to the Mediterranean region, including parts of Europe, Africa, and Asia.

Habitat: This hardy plant grows in dry, rocky soils and can tolerate drought and salt spray. It is often found growing wild on hillsides and in coastal areas.

Plant Parts Used: The leaves and essential oil are the primary parts used medicinally. The leaves are often used in dried or fresh form, while the oil is used in aromatherapy and topical applications.

Therapeutic Properties

Therapeutic Actions:

- *Carminative:* Helps expel gas and relieve bloating
- *Nervine:* Calms and supports the nervous system
- *Nootropic:* Enhances cognitive function and memory
- *Antimicrobial:* Helps fight against bacterial and fungal infections
- *Antioxidant:* Protects cells from damage caused by free radicals

Indications:

- Digestive issues, such as indigestion and bloating
- Stress and anxiety
- Cognitive decline and memory impairment
- Respiratory infections and congestion
- Cardiovascular disorders

Energetics: Rosemary has a warming and drying energy. It is considered a pungent and slightly bitter herb in Western herbalism.

Safety and Dosage

Dosage:

- Infusion: 1–2 teaspoons of dried herb per cup of boiling water, steeped for 10–15 minutes, taken 2–3 times daily
- Tincture: 2–4 mL, taken 2–3 times daily

- Essential oil: 1–2 drops diluted in a carrier oil for topical application or inhalation

Contraindications: Rosemary should be used cautiously by individuals with epilepsy or seizure disorders, as it may potentially trigger seizures in high doses. It should also be avoided by pregnant women, as it may stimulate menstruation.

Interactions: Rosemary may interact with certain medications, such as anticoagulants, diuretics, and lithium. It may also interfere with the absorption of iron and other minerals.

St John's Wort

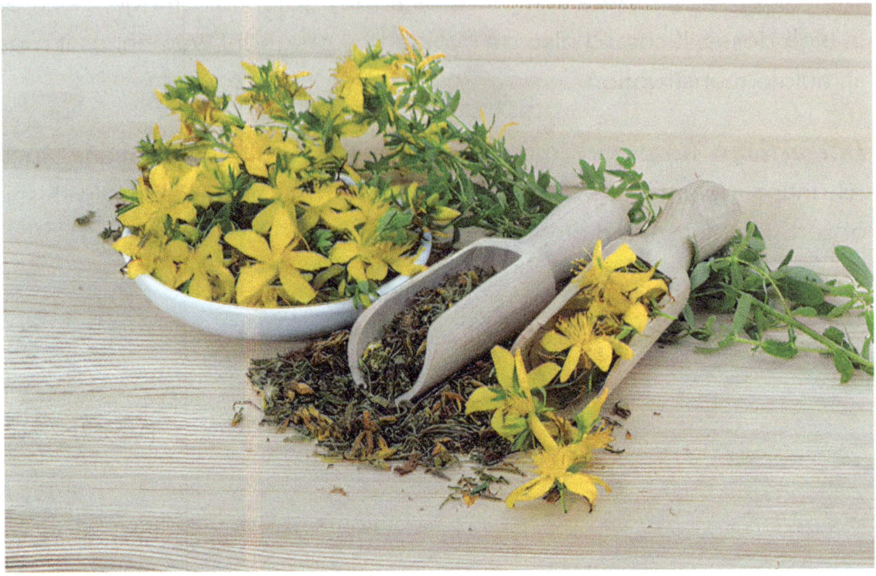

Botanical Information

Scientific Name: *Hypericum perforatum*

Plant Description: St. John's Wort is a perennial herb that typically grows to a height of 30–60 cm. It has opposite, oblong leaves that are covered in tiny, transparent dots. The plant produces bright yellow, star-shaped flowers with five petals.

Native Region: St. John's Wort is native to Europe, North Africa, and parts of Asia but has been naturalized in many other parts of the world, including North America and Australia.

Habitat: This adaptable plant can grow in a variety of habitats, from sunny meadows to dry, rocky soils. It often thrives in disturbed areas and can become invasive in some regions.

Plant Parts Used: The aerial parts (leaves and flowers) are the primary parts used medicinally, often in dried form. The essential oil is also used in some preparations.

Therapeutic Properties

Therapeutic Actions:

- *Antidepressant:* Helps alleviate symptoms of mild to moderate depression
- *Nervine:* Calms and supports the nervous system
- *Astringent:* Tightens and tones tissues, particularly in the digestive tract
- *Vulnerary:* Promotes wound healing and tissue repair
- *Antiviral:* Helps fight against viral infections, particularly herpes and HIV

Indications:

- Mild to moderate depression
- Anxiety and nervous tension
- Digestive issues, such as diarrhea and ulcers
- Skin conditions, such as wounds and burns
- Viral infections, including herpes and HIV

Energetics: St. John's Wort has a cooling and drying energy. It is considered a bitter and pungent herb in Western herbalism.

Safety and Dosage

Dosage:

- Infusion: 1–2 teaspoons of dried herb per cup of boiling water, steeped for 10–15 minutes, taken 2–3 times daily
- Tincture: 2–4 mL, taken 2–3 times daily
- Capsules: 1–2 capsules (300–500 mg), taken 2–3 times daily

Contraindications: St. John's Wort should be avoided by individuals taking certain medications, such as antidepressants, birth control pills, and blood thinners, as it may interact with these drugs. It should also be avoided by pregnant women, as it may stimulate menstruation.

Interactions: St. John's Wort is known to interact with a wide range of medications, including antidepressants, anticoagulants, and immunosuppressants. It may also interfere with the absorption of iron and other minerals and increase the risk of photosensitivity.

Turmeric

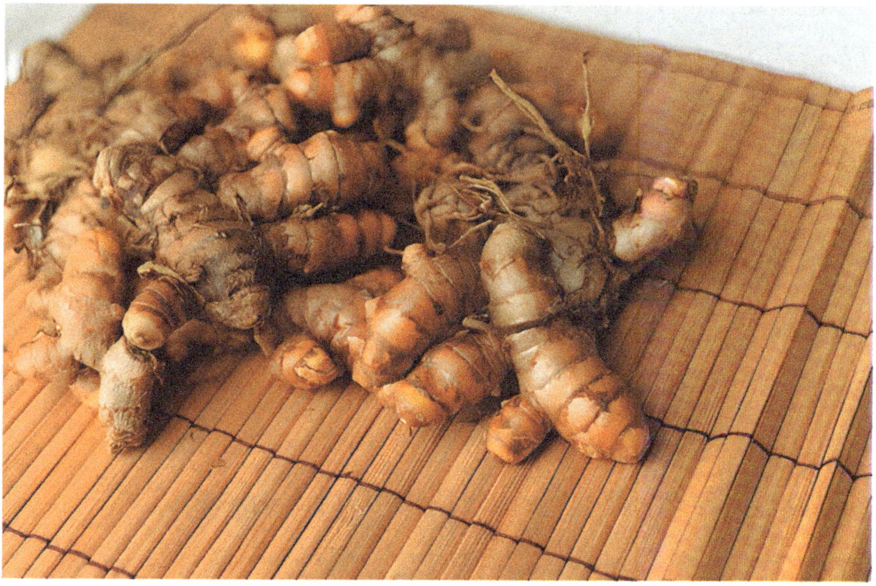

Botanical Information

Scientific Name: *Curcuma longa*

Plant Description: Turmeric is a perennial herb that typically grows to a height of 1–1.5 meters. It has large, lance-shaped leaves and produces pale yellow flowers on a central spike. The plant has a thick, knobbly rhizome that is often bright orange or yellow in color.

Native Region: Turmeric is native to South Asia, particularly India and Indonesia, but is now widely cultivated in tropical regions around the world.

Habitat: This tropical plant thrives in hot, humid climates and prefers well-drained, fertile soils. It is often grown as a cash crop in tropical countries.

Plant Parts Used: The rhizome is the primary part used medicinally and as a culinary spice, often in dried or powdered form.

Therapeutic Properties

Therapeutic Actions:

- *Anti-inflammatory:* Reduces inflammation throughout the body
- *Antioxidant:* Protects cells from damage caused by free radicals
- *Hepatoprotective:* Supports liver health and function
- *Digestive:* Stimulates bile production and aids in digestion
- *Neuroprotective:* May help prevent cognitive decline and neurodegenerative diseases

Indications:

- Inflammatory conditions, such as arthritis and colitis
- Digestive issues, such as indigestion and bloating
- Liver disorders, such as hepatitis and cirrhosis
- Cognitive decline and memory impairment
- Skin conditions, such as eczema and psoriasis

Energetics: Turmeric has a warming and slightly drying energy. It is considered a bitter and pungent herb in Western herbalism.

Safety and Dosage

Dosage:

- Decoction: 1–2 teaspoons of dried rhizome per cup of water, simmered for 10–15 minutes, taken 2–3 times daily
- Tincture: 2–4 mL, taken 2–3 times daily
- Capsules: 1–2 capsules (400–600 mg), taken 2–3 times daily

Contraindications: Turmeric should be used cautiously by individuals with gallstones or bile duct obstruction, as it may stimulate bile production. It should also be avoided by pregnant women in medicinal doses, as it may stimulate uterine contractions.

Interactions: Turmeric may interact with certain medications, such as anticoagulants and antiplatelet drugs, as it may enhance their effects. It may also interfere with the absorption of iron and other minerals.

Valerian

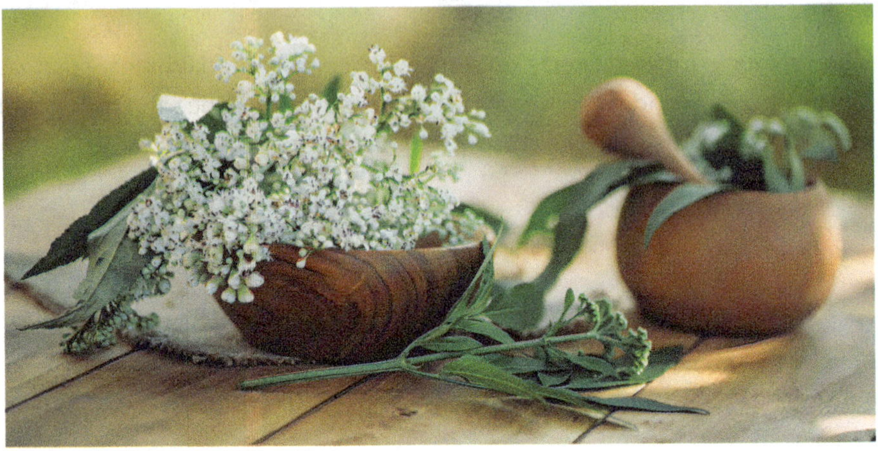

Botanical Information

Scientific Name: *Valeriana officinalis*

Plant Description: Valerian is a perennial herb that typically grows to a height of 1–1.5 meters. It has pinnate, compound leaves and produces small, pink, or white flowers in clusters at the top of the stem. The plant has a thick, fibrous root system that has a strong, earthy odor.

Native Region: Valerian is native to Europe and parts of Asia but has been naturalized in many other parts of the world, including North America.

Habitat: This hardy plant can grow in a variety of habitats, from moist woodlands to dry, rocky soils. It is often found in disturbed areas and can become invasive in some regions.

Plant Parts Used: The roots and rhizomes are the primary parts used medicinally, often in dried or powdered form.

Therapeutic Properties

Therapeutic Actions:

- *Sedative:* Promotes relaxation and aids in sleep
- *Anxiolytic:* Helps to relieve anxiety and nervousness
- *Antispasmodic:* Relieves muscle spasms and tension
- *Hypnotic:* Induces sleep and improves sleep quality
- *Nervine:* Calms and supports the nervous system

Indications:

- Insomnia and sleep disturbances
- Anxiety and nervous tension
- Muscle spasms and tension
- Restlessness and agitation
- Stress and irritability

Energetics: Valerian has a warming and slightly moistening energy. It is considered a pungent and slightly bitter herb in Western herbalism.

Safety and Dosage

Dosage:

- Infusion: 1–2 teaspoons of dried root per cup of boiling water, steeped for 10–15 minutes, taken 30–60 minutes before bedtime
- Tincture: 2–4 mL, taken 30–60 minutes before bedtime
- Capsules: 1–2 capsules (300–600 mg), taken 30–60 minutes before bedtime

Contraindications: Valerian should be used cautiously by individuals with liver disease, as it may impair liver function in high doses. It should also be avoided by pregnant women, as it may stimulate uterine contractions.

Interactions: Valerian may interact with certain medications, such as sedatives, anxiolytics, and anticonvulsants, potentially enhancing their effects. It may also interfere with the absorption of iron and other minerals.

GLOSSARY

Action: The specific effects an herb has on the body.

Adaptogens: Herbs that help the body handle stress.

Alkaloids: Plant compounds containing nitrogen, often with strong effects on the body.

Anti-inflammatory: Herbs that reduce inflammation.

Antioxidants: Compounds that protect cells from damage.

Bioavailability: How well an herb's active compounds can be absorbed and used by the body.

Constituents: The individual compounds within an herb that give it medicinal properties.

Contraindications: Situations where an herb shouldn't be used due to potential harm.

Decoction: An herbal preparation made by simmering tougher plant parts in water.

Endocrine system: Glands that produce hormones to regulate body functions.

Energetics: A traditional way of understanding how herbs affect the body based on their properties.

Flavonoids: Plant compounds known for antioxidant and anti-inflammatory effects.

Glycosides: Plant compounds made of a sugar bound to a non-sugar molecule.

Holistic: An approach that considers the whole person, not just symptoms.

Infusion: An herbal preparation made by steeping herbs in hot water.

Metabolism: The chemical reactions in the body that sustain life.

Phytochemicals: The various bioactive compounds found in plants.

Polysaccharides: Complex carbohydrate molecules found in many medicinal plants.

Synergy: When the combined effect of an herb's compounds is greater than the sum of their individual effects.

Terpenes: A diverse class of aromatic plant compounds, many with medicinal properties.

Tincture: A concentrated liquid extract of an herb, usually made with alcohol.

Wildcrafting: Harvesting medicinal plants from their natural habitats.

RESOURCES

This resources section provides a curated list of trusted resources to support your herbal journey. As you explore these resources, remember to approach new information with a critical eye and evaluate the credibility of sources. By incorporating these tools into your herbal education, you'll be well-equipped to make informed decisions and continue growing in your practice.

Herbal Suppliers

Mountain Rose Herbs: A leading supplier for organic herbs, spices, and herbal products. Known for their sustainable practices, they offer a wide selection of dried herbs, teas, and other herbal remedies. (**http://www.mountainroseherbs.com/**)

Pacific Botanicals: They specialize in fresh and dried organic herbs with a commitment to regenerative farming practices. Their offerings include rare and wildcrafted herbs.

Starwest Botanicals: Providing a vast range of organic and wildcrafted herbs, essential oils, and herbal extracts, they are a go-to supplier for many herbalists. (**http://www.starwest-botanicals.com/**)

Frontier Natural Products Co-Op: A member-owned cooperative offering a wide selection of organic and sustainably sourced herbs, spices, and herbal products. (**http://www.frontiercoop.com/**)

Healing Spirits Herb Farm & Education Center: A family-owned farm and education center offering organically grown and ethically wildcrafted herbs, along with herbal workshops and classes. (**http://www.healingspiritsherbfarm.com/**)

Jean's Greens: Specializing in organic and wildcrafted herbs, teas, and herbal products, with a focus on sustainability and quality. (**http://www.jeansgreens.com/**)

Wild Weeds: Offering a unique selection of wildcrafted and organically grown herbs, with an emphasis on bioregional and sustainable sourcing. (**http://www.wildweeds.com/**)

Zack Woods Herb Farm: A small, family-owned herb farm offering organically grown and ethically wildcrafted herbs with a commitment to sustainable practices and education. (**http://www.zackwoodsherbs.com/**)

Acorn School of Herbal Medicine: In addition to offering educational programs, Acorn School of Herbal Medicine provides a selection of high-quality, ethically wildcrafted or organically cultivated herbs. They prioritize working with local farmers and wildcrafters to ensure sustainability and freshness. (**http://www.acornherbschool.com/herbal-supplies**)

Herbal Products

Wise Woman Herbals: Offering a wide range of herbal extracts, tinctures, and capsules crafted using organic and wildcrafted herbs. (**http://www.wisewomanherbals.com/**)

Gaia Herbs: Known for their high-quality, potent herbal extracts and supplements, with a commitment to transparency and sustainability. (**http://www.gaiaherbs.com/**)

Avena Botanicals: A small, woman-owned company offering handcrafted herbal remedies, including tinctures, salves, and teas. (**http://www.avenaherbs.com/**)

Empowered Herbals: Specializing in herbal syrups and elixirs, crafted using organic and wildcrafted herbs, with a focus on sustainable and ethical sourcing. (**http://www.empoweredherbals.com/**)

Equinox Botanicals: Offering a range of herbal tinctures, oils, and salves crafted using organic and ethically wildcrafted herbs. (https://equinoxbotanicals.com/)

Herb Pharm: A leading provider of high-quality, potent herbal extracts and tinctures with a commitment to sustainable and ethical sourcing. (http://www.herb-pharm.com/)

Herbalist & Alchemist: Offering a wide range of herbal tinctures, oils, and other remedies, crafted using traditional herbal methods and organic or wildcrafted herbs. (http://www.herbalist-alchemist.com/)

Traditional Medicinals: Known for their high-quality, medicinal-grade herbal teas and supplements, with a focus on sustainability and social responsibility. (http://www.traditionalmedicinals.com/)

Sage Mountain Herb Products: Offering a range of herbal remedies, including tinctures, oils, and salves, crafted by renowned herbalist Rosemary Gladstar. (http://www.healingspiritsherbfarm.com/)

Simpler's Botanical Company: Specializing in herbal extracts and tinctures crafted using organic and wildcrafted herbs, with a commitment to quality and sustainability. (http://www.simplers.com/)

Woodland Essence: Offering a range of herbal remedies, including tinctures, salves, and teas, crafted using organic and ethically wildcrafted herbs. (http://www.woodlandessence.com/)

Plant Identification Apps

PlantSnap: An easy-to-use app that helps identify plants, flowers, and trees using AI. It's a great tool for beginners.

Seek by iNaturalist: A reliable app that identifies plants and animals in real-time using your phone's camera. Developed by National Geographic and the California Academy of Sciences.

PictureThis: A widely-used app that provides plant identification through photos with a high level of accuracy.

Community Platforms

HerbMentor: An online community with courses and forums where herbalists of all levels can share experiences and knowledge.

The Herbal Academy's Herbarium: A membership-based resource offering a wealth of information, herbal monographs, and community engagement opportunities for herbal enthusiasts. (http://www.theherbalacademy.com/)

Education and Training

Acorn School of Herbal Medicine: Offering a variety of online and in-person herbal medicine courses, workshops, and apprenticeships. (http://www.acornherbschool.com/)

North American Institute of Medical Herbalism (NAIMH): Providing comprehensive herbal medicine education, including online courses and a clinical herbalist diploma program. (http://www.naimh.com/)

The Herbal Academy: Offering a wide range of online herbal courses, from beginner to advanced levels, with a focus on practical skills and holistic healing. (http://www.theherbalacademy.com/herbalism-courses)

ArborVitae School of Traditional Herbalism: Based in New York City, offering in-person and online herbal medicine courses, workshops, and certification programs. (http://www.arborvitaeny.com/)

American Herb Association: A non-profit organization dedicated to promoting the use of herbs and herbal education. (http://www.ahaherb.com/)

United States American Herbalists Guild: A professional association of herbal practitioners that provides educational resources, conferences, and a directory of qualified herbalists. (http://www.americanherbalist.com/)

California School of Herbal Studies: Offering a variety of herbal medicine courses, workshops, and certification programs, with a focus on traditional Western herbalism. (http://www.cshs.com/)

Herb Research Foundation: A non-profit organization dedicated to supporting research on the safety and efficacy of herbal medicine. (http://www.herbs.org/)

Mountain Rose Herbals: In addition to their herbal products, Mountain Rose Herbals offers a variety of educational resources, including articles, videos, and workshops. (http://www.mountainroseherbs.com/herbal-education)

Sage Mountain Retreat Center & Botanical Sanctuary: Founded by Rosemary Gladstar, offering herbal education programs, workshops, and retreats in a beautiful Vermont setting. (http://www.sagemountain.com/)

Herbal Information

The Herbarium: A comprehensive online database of herbal monographs, providing detailed information on the properties, uses, and safety of over 150 herbs. (http://www.theherbalacademy.com/)

The Naturopathic Herbalist: A website offering a wide range of articles and resources on herbal medicine, nutrition, and natural health. (http://www.thenaturopathicherbalist.com/)

United Plant Savers: A non-profit organization dedicated to protecting native medicinal plants and their habitats, offering education and resources for sustainable herbalism. (**http://www.unitedplantsavers.org/**)

Henriette's Herbal Homepage: A comprehensive collection of herbal resources, including articles, book excerpts, and a forum for herbal enthusiasts. (**http://www.henriettes-herb.com/**)

Journals

Medical Herbalism: A quarterly journal featuring articles on herbal medicine, case studies, and book reviews. (**http://www.medherb.com/articles.htm**)

The Essential Herbal: A bimonthly magazine featuring articles on herbal medicine, recipes, and crafts. (**http://www.essentialherbal.com/**)

Journal of Herbs, Spices & Medical Plants: A peer-reviewed journal publishing research on the cultivation, processing, and use of herbs and spices for medicinal purposes. (**http://www.tandfonline.com/toc/whsm20/30/4**)

Journal of Medicinal Herbs: An international, peer-reviewed journal publishing original research articles, reviews, and short communications on medicinal herbs. (**http://www.sanad.iau.ir/journal/jhd**)

Garden Troubleshooting

Local Agricultural Extension Offices: These offices, often affiliated with state universities, provide a wealth of resources and expertise for gardeners and farmers. They can help with identifying specific pests or diseases affecting your herbs and provide tailored advice for your local growing conditions. Find your local extension office here: (**http://www.almanac.com/content/cooperative-extension-services**)

Master Gardener Programs: These programs, also often affiliated with local extension offices, consist of trained volunteers who can offer gardening advice and troubleshooting. Find a Master Gardener program near you: (**https://mastergardener.extension.org/**)

Local Gardening Clubs or Organizations: Connecting with other herb gardeners in your area can provide a great opportunity to share knowledge and learn from others' experiences. Search for local gardening clubs or organizations in your area.

Online Gardening Forums and Communities: Many online platforms host active communities of gardeners where you can ask questions, share photos, and get advice from experienced growers. Some popular forums include:

- GardenWeb: http://www.houzz.com/
- Dave's Garden: http://www.davesgarden.com/
- Permies: http://www.permies.com/

Plant Disease and Pest Diagnostic Clinics: Some universities and agricultural organizations offer diagnostic services where you can send in samples of affected plants for identification and treatment recommendations. Check with your local extension office or university for available services.

REFERENCES

Akhondzadeh, S., Naghavi, H. R., Vazirian, M., Shayeganpour, A., Rashidi, H., & Khani, M. (2002). Passionflower in the treatment of generalized anxiety disorder: A systematic review. Journal of Clinical Pharmacy and Therapeutics, 26(5), 363–367. https://doi.org/10.1046/j.1365-2710.2001.00367.x

Bent, S., & Ko, R. (2004). Commonly used herbal medicines in the United States: A review. *American Journal of Medicine*, *116*(7), 478–485. https://doi.org/10.1016/j.amjmed.2003.10.036

Blessing, E. M., Steenkamp, M. M., Manzanares, J., & Marmar, C. R. (2015). Cannabidiol as a potential treatment for anxiety disorders. *Neurotherapeutics*, *12*(4), 825-836. https://doi.org/10.1007/s13311-015-0387-1

Bone, K., & Mills, S. (2013). *Principles and practice of phytotherapy: Modern herbal medicine* (2nd ed.). Churchill Livingstone Elsevier.

Borchers, A. T., Keen, C. L., Stern, J. S., & Gershwin, M. E. (2000). Inflammation and Native American medicine: The role of botanicals. *The American Journal of Clinical Nutrition*, *72*(2), 339–347. https://doi.org/10.1093/ajcn/72.2.339_

Chan, Y.S., Cheng, L. N., Wu, J. H., Chan, E., Kwan, Y.W., Lee, S. M. Y., Leung, G. P. H., Yu, P. H. F., & Chan, S.-W. (2010). A review of the pharmacological effects of Arctium lappa (burdock). *Inflammopharmacology*, *19*, 245–254. https://doi.org/10.1007/s10787-010-0062-4

Cheng, Y.-C., Li, T. S., Su, H. L., Lee, P. C., & Wang, H.-M. D. (2020). Transdermal Delivery Systems of Natural Products Applied to Skin Therapy and Care. *Molecules (Basel, Switzerland)*, *25*(21), 5051. https://doi.org/10.3390/molecules25215051

Cohen, M. M. (2014). Tulsi - Ocimum sanctum: A herb for all reasons. *Journal of Ayurveda and Integrative Medicine, 5*(4), 251–259. **https://pubmed.ncbi.nlm.nih.gov/25624701/**

Cohen, R. A., Kucera, L. S., & Herrmann, E. C. (1964). Antiviral Activity of Melissa officinalis (Lemon Balm) Extract. *Experimental Biology and Medicine, 117*(2), 431–434. **https://doi.org/10.3181/00379727-117-29600**

Coulter, I. D., Herman, P. M., & Nataraj, S. (2013). Economic analysis of complementary, alternative, and integrative medicine: considerations raised by an expert panel. *BMC Complementary and Alternative Medicine, 13*(1), 191. **https://doi.org/10.1186/1472-6882-13-191**

Dai, Y.-L., Li, Y., Wang, Q., Niu, F.-J., Li, K.-W., Wang, Y.-Y., Wang, J., Zhou, C.-Z., & Gao, L.-N. (2022). Chamomile: A review of its traditional uses, chemical constituents, pharmacological activities, and quality control studies. *Molecules, 28*(1), 133. **https://doi.org/10.3390/molecules28010133**

Efferth, T., & Koch, E. (2011). Complex interactions between phytochemicals: The multi-target therapeutic concept of phytotherapy. *Current Drug Targets, 12*(1), 122–132. **https://doi.org/10.2174/138945011793591626**

Ekor, M. (2013). The growing use of herbal medicines: Issues relating to adverse reactions and challenges in monitoring safety. *Frontiers in Pharmacology, 4*(177). **https://doi.org/10.3389/fphar.2013.00177**

Foster, S., & Johnson, R. (2006). Desk reference to nature's medicine: The ultimate guide to the best herbs, vitamins, and supplements for your health. National Geographic.

Franco, L., Sánchez, C., Bravo, R., Rodriguez, A., Barriga, C., & Juánez, J. (2012). The sedative effects of hops (Humulus lupulus), a component of beer, on the activity/rest rhythm. *Acta Physiologica Hungarica, 99*(2), 133–139. **https://doi.org/10.1556/aphysiol.99.2012.2.6**

Hewlings, S. J., & Kalman, D. S. (2017). Curcumin: A Review of Its' Effects on Human Health. *Foods, 6*(10), 92. **https://doi.org/10.3390/foods6100092**

Ishaque, S., Shamseer, L., Bukutu, C., & Vohra, S. (2012). Rhodiola rosea for physical and mental fatigue: a systematic review. *BMC Complementary and Alternative Medicine, 12,* 70. **https://doi.org/10.1186/1472-6882-12-70_**

Jurenka, J. S. (2009). Anti-inflammatory properties of curcumin, a major constituent of *Curcuma longa*: A review of preclinical and clinical research. *Alternative Medicine Review, 14*(2), 141–153. **https://pubmed.ncbi.nlm.nih.gov/19594223/**

Khanna, R., MacDonald, J. K., & Levesque, B. G. (2014). Peppermint oil for the treatment of irritable bowel syndrome: A systematic review and meta-analysis. *Journal of Clinical Gastroenterology, 48*(6), 505–512. **https://pubmed.ncbi.nlm.nih.gov/24100754/**

Laakmann, G., Schüle, C., Baghai, T., Kieser, M.(1998). St. John's Wort in mild to moderate depression. *Phytomedicine*, 1, 54–59. **https://pubmed.ncbi.nlm.nih.gov/9684948/**

Li, Y., Pham, V., Bui, M., Song, L., Wu, C., Walia, A., Uchio, E., Smith-Liu, F., & Zi, X. (2017). Rhodiola rosea L.:an herb with anti-stress, anti-aging, and immunostimulating properties for cancer chemoprevention. *Current Pharmacology Reports, 3,* 384–395. **https://doi.org/10.1007/s40495-017-0106-1**

Linde, K., Berner, M. M., & Kriston, L. (2008). St John's wort for major depression. *Cochrane Database of Systematic Reviews, 4.* **https://doi.org/10.1002/14651858.cd000448.pub3**

Lynch, S. V., & Pedersen, O. (2016). The human intestinal microbiome in health and disease. *New England Journal of Medicine, 375*(24), 2369-2379. **https://doi.org/10.1056/NEJMra1600266**

Metwaly, A. M., Ghoneim, M. M., Eissa, I. H., Elsehemy, I. A., Mostafa, A. E., Hegazy, M. M., Afifi, W. M., & Dou, D. (2021). Traditional ancient Egyptian medicine: A review. *Saudi Journal of Biological Sciences, 28*(10), 5823–5832. **https://doi.org/10.1016/j.sjbs.2021.06.044**

Niemeyer, K., Bell, I. R., & Koithan, M. (2013). Traditional knowledge of Western herbal medicine and complex systems science. *Journal of Herbal Medicine, 3*(3), 112–119. **https://pmc.ncbi.nlm.nih.gov/articles/PMC3777424/**

Onyambu, M. O., Gikonya, N.K., Nyambaka, H.N., & Thoithi, G.N. (2019). A Review of Trends in Herbal Drugs Standardization, Regulation and Integration to the National Healthcare Systems in Kenya and the Globe. *International Journal of Pharmacognosy & Chinese Medicine, 3*(3), 1–13. **https://doi.org/10.23880/ipcm-16000168**

Pan, S. Y., Litscher, G., Gao, S. H., Zhou, S. F., Yu, Z. L., Chen, H. Q., Zhang, S. F., Tang, M. K., Sun, J. N., & Ko, K. M. (2014). Historical perspective of traditional indigenous medical practices: The current renaissance and conservation of herbal resources. *Evidence-Based Complementary and Alternative Medicine, 2014*(525340), 1–20. **https://doi.org/10.1155/2014/525340**

Pandey, M. M., Rastogi, S., & Rawat, A. K. S. (2013). Indian traditional Ayurvedic system of medicine and nutritional supplementation. *Evidence-Based Complementary and Alternative Medicine, 2013*, 1–12. **https://doi.org/10.1155/2013/376327**

Panossian, A., & Wikman, G. (2010). Effects of adaptogens on the central nervous system and the molecular mechanisms associated with their stress-protective activity. *Pharmaceuticals, 3*(1), 188–224. **https://doi.org/10.3390/ph3010188**

Petkova, N., Hambarliyska, I., Tumbarski, Y., & Vrancheva, R., Raeva, M., & Ivanov, I. (2021). Phytochemical Composition and Antimicrobial Properties of Burdock (Arctium lappa L.) Roots Extracts. *Biointerface*

Research in Applied Chemistry, 12(3), 2826–2842. https://doi.org/10.33263/briac123.28262842

Ryan, J. L., Heckler, C. E., Roscoe, J. A., Dakhil, S. R., Kirshner, J., Flynn, P. J., Hickok, J. T., & Morrow, G. R. (2011). Ginger (*Zingiber officinale*) reduces acute chemotherapy-induced nausea: A URCC CCOP study of 576 patients. *Supportive Care in Cancer, 20*(7), 1479–1489. https://doi.org/10.1007/s00520-011-1236-3

Sustainable Herbs Initiative. (n.d.). What are sustainable herbs? *Sustainable Herbs Initiative.* https://sustainableherbsinitiative.org/explore/what-is-sustainable-medicine/

Thomford, N. E., Dzobo, K., Chimusa, E., Andrae-Marobela, K., Chirikure, S., Wonkam, A., & Dandara, C. (2018). Personalized Herbal Medicine? A Roadmap for Convergence of Herbal and Precision Medicine Biomarker Innovations. *OMICS: A Journal of Integrative Biology, 22*(6), 375–391. https://doi.org/10.1089/omi.2018.0074

Tiralongo, E., Wee, S. S., & Lea, R. A. (2016). Elderberry supplementation reduces cold duration and symptoms in air travelers: A randomized, double-blind placebo-controlled clinical trial. *Nutrients, 8*(4), 182. https://pubmed.ncbi.nlm.nih.gov/27023596/

Ulbricht, C., Basch, E., Cheung, L., Goldberg, H., Hammerness, P., Isaac, R., Khalsa, K. P., Romm, A., Rychlik, I., & Varghese, M., Weissmer, W., Windsor, C. R., & Wortley, J. (2014). An evidence-based systematic review of elderberry and elderflower (*Sambucus nigra*) by the Natural Standard Research Collaboration. *Journal of Dietary Supplements, 11*(1), 80–120. https://pubmed.ncbi.nlm.nih.gov/24409980/

Wahab, S., Annadurai, S., Abullais, S. S., Das, G., Ahmad, W., Ahmad, M. F., Kandasamy, G., Vasudevan, R., Ali, M. S., & Amir, M. (2021). Glycyrrhiza glabra (Licorice): A Comprehensive Review on Its Phytochemistry, Biological Activities, Clinical Evidence and Toxicology. *Plants, 10*(12), 2751. https://doi.org/10.3390/plants10122751

Wang, L., Waltenberger, B., Pferschy-Wenzig, E.-M., Blunder, M., Liu, X., Malainer, C., Blazevic, T., Schwaiger, S., Rollinger, J. M., Heiss, E. H., Schuster, D., Kopp, B., Bauer, R., Stuppner, H., Dirsch, V. M., & Atanasov, A. G. (2014). Natural product agonists of peroxisome proliferator-activated receptor gamma (PPARγ): a review. *Biochemical Pharmacology, 92*(1), 73–89. https://doi.org/10.1016/j.bcp.2014.07.018

Weber, W., Taylor, J. A., Stoep, A. V., Weiss, N. S., Standish, L. J., & Calabrese, C. (2005). Echinacea purpurea for Prevention of Upper Respiratory Tract Infections in Children. *The Journal of Alternative and Complementary Medicine, 11*(6), 1021–1026. https://doi.org/10.1089/acm.2005.11.1021

Williamson, E. M. (2001). Synergy and other interactions in phytomedicines. *Phytomedicine, 8*(5), 401–409. https://doi.org/10.1078/0944-7113-00060

Wilms, S. (2017). The divine farmer's classic of materia medica = Shén nóng běncǎo jīng. Happy Goat Productions.

Zhou, S., Lim, L. Y., & Chowbay, B. (2004). Herbal Modulation of P-Glycoprotein. *Drug Metabolism Reviews, 36*(1), 57–104. https://doi.org/10.1081/dmr-120028427

INDEX

B

D

E

F

G

H

I

L

M

N

Q

R

S

T

Made in the USA
Monee, IL
03 November 2026

67377195R00148